The Middle English Ideal of Personal Beauty

AMS PRESS
NEW YORK

The Middle English Ideal of Personal Beauty; as Found in the Metrical Romances, Chronicles, and Legends of the XIII, XIV, and XV Centuries.

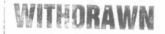

BY

WALTER CLYDE CURRY
Instructor in English, Vanderbilt University

BALTIMORE
J. H. FURST COMPANY
1916

Library of Congress Cataloging in Publication Data

Curry, Walter Clyde, 1887-1967.
   The Middle English ideal of personal beauty.

   Originally presented as the author's thesis,
Stanford, 1915.
   Bibliography: p.
   1. English poetry--Middle English (1100-1500)
--History and criticism. 2. Beauty, Personal, in
literature. I. Title.
PR317.B4C8 1972   821'.1'09353   72-000010
ISBN 0-404-01886-6

PR
317
B4
C8
1972

Reprinted from the edition of 1916, Baltimore
First AMS edition published in 1972
Manufactured in the United States of America

International Standard Book Number: 0-404-01886-6

AMS PRESS INC.
NEW YORK, N. Y.   10003

PREFACE

In May of 1915 this study was presented to the Faculty of Arts and Sciences of Leland Stanford Junior University in partial fulfillment of the requirements for the degree of Doctor of Philosophy. It is now being published in the hope that it may throw some light on the customs and manners of the English people of the thirteenth, fourteenth, and fifteenth centuries, on the entirely conventional habits of thought and expression as found in the literature of the time, and on the debt of Middle English literature to other literatures of medieval times. Within the restricted limits of the field of research, my prime object, both in the collection and in the presentation of material, has been thoroness and accuracy; so that those who may be interested in this particular subject may find here a reasonably trustworthy work of reference.

I gratefully acknowledge my indebtedness to the authorities of the University, and my specific obligations to Professors H. D. Gray, O. M. Johnston, and Dr. A. G. Kennedy, and especially to Professor R. M. Alden, under whose direction this dissertation was completed, for his sympathetic advice and invaluable suggestions. I wish also to pay high tribute to the inspiring example of sound scholarship and patient and penetrating criticism of my master, the late Doctor Ewald Flügel, under whose guidance this work was begun and almost finished.

WALTER CLYDE CURRY.

Vanderbilt University, October, 1916.

TABLE OF CONTENTS

	PAGE
INTRODUCTION	1
HAIR	11
BEARD	35
FOREHEAD	42
EYEBROWS	44
EYES	51
NOSE; NOSTRILS	63
EARS	65
MOUTH, LIPS, BREATH	66
TONGUE	69
TEETH, GUMS	69
VOICE	71
CHIN	73
FACE; COUNTENANCE	74
SKIN; SKIN OF FACE	80
CHEEKS; COMPLEXION	91
HEAD	99
NECK	99
FORM, FIGURE, STATURE	101
SHOULDERS	111
BREAST; BREASTS	112
BACK	114
SIDES; WAIST	114
ABDOMEN	116
LOINS; HIPS	117
LIMBS; BONES	118
ARMS	121
HANDS; FINGERS; FIST	122
LEGS	124
FEET	126

BIBLIOGRAPHY AND ABBREVIATIONS.

ROMANCES.

Adler.	Kinge Adler, ed. J. W. Hales and F. J. Furnivall, *Percy Folio MS.* Lon. 1867-8, Vol. II, 269 ff.
Alis A.	Alisaunder, ed. W. W. Skeat, EETS. 1, 1890.
Alis B.	Alexander and Dindemus, ed. W. W. Skeat, EETS. E. S. 31, 1878.
Alis C.	The Wars of Alexander, ed. W. W. Skeat, EETS. E. S. 47.
Alis L.	Alisaunder, ed. Weber, *Metrical Romances*, Edin. 1810, Vol. I.
Amad.	Sir Amadace, ed. J. Robson, *Three Early English Metrical Romances*, Camden Society, 1842.
Am & Am.	Amis and Amiloun, ed. E. Koelbing, *Alteng. Bibliothek*, Heil. 1884, Vol. II.
Arth.	Arthur, ed. Furnivall, EETS. 2, 1868-9.
Arth. & Merl.	Arthur and Merlin, ed. E. Koelbing, Alteng. Bibl. Vol. IV. 1890.
Chev. Assig.	Cheulere Assigne, ed. H. G. Gibbs, EETS. E. S. 6, 1868.
Athel.	Athelstan, ed Zupitza, *Eng. Studien*, Vol. XIII. p. 331.
Awn. Arth.	The Awntyrs of Arthure, ed. F. J. Amours, *Scottish Alliterative Poems*, Scot. Text Soc. 1897.
Avow. Arth.	The Avowing of Arthur, ed. Robson, *Three Early Eng. Rom.* 1842.
Beryn.	The Tale of Beryn, ed. Furnivall and Stone, EETS. E. S. 105.
Bev.	Sir Beuis of Hamtoun, ed. Koelbing, EETS. E. S. 46, 48, 60, 1885.
Bon. Flor.	Le Bone Florence of Rome, ed. Ritson, *Ancient English Metrical Romances*, London, 1802, Vol. III. p. 1 ff. Notes, p. 340 ff.
Cleges	Sir Cleges, ed. Weber, *Met. Rom.* Vol. I. 1810.
Degrev.	Sir Degrevant, ed. Halliwell, *Thornton Romances*, Camden Society, 1844.
Dest. Tr.	The 'Geste Hystoriale' of the Destruction of Troy, ed. G. A. Panton and D. Donaldson, EETS. O. S. 39, 56. 1869, 1874.
Eger & Gr.	Eger and Grine, ed. Hales and Furnivall, *Percy Fol. MS.* Vol. I. also ed. Laing, *Early Popular Poetry of Scotland*, Vol. II. 1895.
Eglam.	Sir Aglamour of Artois, ed. G. Schleich, *Palæstra*, Vol. LIII. 1906.
Erl. Tol.	The Erl of Toulous, ed. G. Luedtke, Berlin, 1881.
Emar.	Emaré, ed. E. Rickart, EETS. E. S. 99, Lon. 1906.

Ercel.	Thomas of Erceldoune, ed. J. A. H. Murray, EETS. 61, Lon. 1875.
Ferum.	Sir Ferumbras, ed. S. J. Herrtage, EETS. E. S. 34, Lon. 1879.
Fl. & Bl.	Floriz and Blanchefleur, ed. McKnight, EETS. O. S. Lon. 1901, Vol. 14.
Gaw. & Gr. Kn.	Sir Gawain and the Green Knight, ed. R. Morris, EETS. O. S. 4, 1864-9.
Gam.	Gamelyn, ed. W. W. Skeat, Oxford, 1884.
Gol. & Gaw.	Golagrus and Gawain, ed. F. J. Amours for Scot. Text Soc. 1897.
Gowth.	Sir Gowther, ed. Breul, Berlin, 1883.
Gower	Confessio Amantis, Gower, ed. G. C. Macaulay, 1901.
Guy A.	Guy of Warwick (MS. Auch.), ed. J. Zupitza, EETS. E. S. 42, 49, 59; Guy B. (MS. Cambr.), EETS. E. S. 25, 26; Guy C. (MS. Caius), EETS. E. S. 42, 49, 59.
Grail	Lovelich's "History of the Holy Grail," ed. Furnivall, EETS. E. S. 20, 24, 28, 30, 1874-8; Part v, ed. D. Kempe, EETS. E. S. 95, 1905.
Horn	King Horn, ed. G. H. McKnight, EETS. O. S. 14, 1901.
Havel.	Havelok, ed. Skeat, EETS. E. S. IV. 1867. (Holthausen, *Alt- und mitteleng. Texte* also used.)
Horn Ch.	Horn Child and Maiden Rimnild, ed. J. Caro, *Eng. Stud.* XII. 322.
Iw. & Gw.	Iwain and Gawain, ed. Ritson, *Anc. Eng. Met. Rom.* 1802, Vol. I.
Isum.	Sir Isumbras, ed. Zupitza and Schleich, *Palæstra*, XV. 1901.
Ipom.	Ipomedon, ed. Koelbing, Breslau, 1889.
Jos. Arim.	Joseph of Arimathie, ed. W. W. Skeat, EETS. E. S. 44, 1871.
Kn. of Cour.	The Knight of Courtesy, ed. Ritson, *A. E. M. R.* Vol. III. 1802.
Lancel.	Lancelot of the Laik, ed. Skeat, EETS. O. S. 6, 1865.
Launf. M.	Launfal Miles, ed. Kaluza, *Engl. Stud.* XVIII, 165.
Launf. R.	Landavall, ed. G. L. Kittredge, *Amer. Journal of Philology*, Vol. X.
Lib. Des.	Libeaus Desconus, ed. Kaluza, *Alteng. Bibl.* Vol. V. 1890.
Lyd.	Lydgate's Troy Book, ed. H. Bergen, EETS. E. S. 97, 106, 193, 1906.
Mort. Arth.	Morte Arthure, ed. G. G. Perry, EETS. O. S. 8, 1865.
Le Mort. Arth.	Le Morte Arthur, ed. J. D. Bruce, EETS. E. S. 88, 1903.
Orph.	Sir Orpheo (MS. Harl.), ed. Ritson, *A. E. M. R.* Vol. II.
Orf.	Sir Orfeo, ed. Zielke (MS. Auch.); ed. Laing, *Early Popular Poetry of Scotland*, Vol. I.
Otuel	Otuel, ed. Herrtage, EETS. E. S. 39, 1882.
Oct S.	Octavian (Southern version); Octavian (Northern Version), ed. G. Sarrazin, *Altengl. Bibl.* Vol. III. 1885.

Parton.	Partonope of Blois, ed. Boedtker, EETS. E. S. 109, 1912.
Perc. Gal.	Sir Percival of Galles, ed. Campion and Holthausen, Heidelb. 1913.
Pist. Sus.	The Pistill of Susan, ed. Amours, Scot. Text Soc. 27, 38, 1892-97.
Rich.	Richard Coeur de Lion, ed. Weber, *Met. Rom.* 1810, Vol. II.
Rol. & Ot.	Roland and Otuel, ed. Herrtage, EETS. E. S. 35, 1881.
Rol. & Vern.	Roland and Vernagu, ed. Herrtage, EETS. E. S. 39, 1882.
Sev. Sag.	Seven Sages, ed. Weber, *Met. Rom.* 1810, Vol. III.
Sow. Bab.	The Sowdowne of Babylone, ed. E. Hausknecht, EETS. E. S. 38.
Sege Mel.	The Sege of Melayne, ed. Herrtage, EETS. E. S. 35, 1880.
Song Rol.	The Song of Roland, ed. Herrtage, EETS. E. S. 35, 1880.
Squyr.	The Squyr of Lowe Degre, ed. Ritson, *A. E. M. R.* 1802, Vol. III.
Tars.	The King of Tars, ed. F. Krause, *Engl. Stud.* XI.
Torr.	Torrent of Portyngale, ed. E. Adam, EETS. E. S. 51, 1887.
Triam.	Sir Triamour, ed. J. O. Halliwell, Percy Society, XVI. 1846.
Troy B.	Seege of Troye, ed. A. Zietsch, in Herrig's *Archiv*, 72; Troy H. (MS. Harl.), *ibid.*
Trist.	Sir Tristrem, ed. Koelbing, Heilbronn, 1878.
Wm. Pal.	William of Palerne, ed. Skeat, EETS. E. S. I. 1832, 1867.
Wed. Gaw.	The Weddynge of Sir Gawen and Dame Ragnell (frag.), ed. Hales and Furnivall, *Percy Fol. MS.* Vol. I.

LYRICS.

Boedd.	*Altenglische Dichtungen des MS. Harl. 2253,* ed. Boeddeker, Berlin, 1878.
Lob. Frau.	*Lob der Frauen,* ed. Koelbing, *Engl. Stud.* VII.
Max.	Maximion, ed. Boeddeker, in *Altengl. Dicht. d. MS. Harl. 2253.* Berlin, 1873.

LEGEND.

Boc.	Osbern Bockenam's *Legenden,* ed. Horstmann, C., in *Altengl. Bibl.* Vol. I, Heilb. 1883.
Cur. Mun.	Cursor Mundi, ed. R. Morris, EETS. O. S. 57, 59, 62, 66, 68, 69, 101. 1874-93.
Gregor.	Die Gregoriuslegende, ed. C. Keller, in *Alt- und Mittel-eng. Texte,* Vol. VI, 1914.
Horst A.	Altenglische Legenden, ed. C. Horstmann, Paderborn, 1895.
Horst B.	Altenglische Legenden, ed. Horstmann, Heilbronn, 1878.

x   *Bibliography and Abbreviations*

Horst C.	Altenglische Legenden, Neue Folge, ed. Horstmann, Heilbronn, 1881.
Horst D.	Early South English Legendary, ed. Horstmann, EETS. O. S. 87. 1887.
Marh.	Seinte Marherete, ed. O. Cockayne, EETS. O. S. 13, 1866.
Sc. Leg.	Scottish Légends of the Saints, ed. W. M. Metcalfe, for Scot. Text Soc. 1896.

CHRONICLES.

Barb.	Barbour's Bruce, ed Skeat, for Scot. Text Soc. 1894. (also for EETS. 1870-89.)
R. Brunn.	Robert of Brunne's Chornicle of England, ed. Furnivall, Rolls Series, No. 87, 1887.
Conq. Ire.	The Conquest of Ireland, ed. Furnivall, EETS. O. S. 107, 1896.
Gir. Cam.	Giraldus Cambrensis, *Opera*, Rolls Series, No. 21, 8 vols. ed. (Vols. I-VI.) J. S. Brewer; Vol. VII, J. F. Dimock; Vol. VIII, G. F. Warner.
Geof. Mon.	Geoffrey of Monmouth, *Historia Regum Britanniae*, ed. San Marte, Halle, 1854. (Trans. G. A. Giles, *Six Old English Chronicles*.)
Hen. Hunt.	Henry of Huntington, *Historia Anglorum*, ed. Thos. Arnold, Rolls Series, No. 74, 1879. (Trans. Thos. Forester, 1853.)
Hig-Trev.	Higden-Trevisa, *Polychronicon*, ed. C. Babington, Rolls Series, No. 41, 1865-79. 9 vols.
Joc. Brak.	Jocelin de Brakelond, *Cronica*, ed. J. G. Rokewode for Camden Soc. 1840.
Laȝ.	Laȝamon's Brut, ed. F. Madden, Lon. 1847.
Pier. Lang.	Robert of Brunne's translation of Pierre de Langtoft's Chronicle of England, ed. Thos. Hearne.
R. Glouc.	The Metrical Chronicle of Robert of Gloucester, ed. W. A. Wright, Rolls Series, No. 86, 1887.
Wm. Malms.	William of Malmsbury, *Gesta Regum Anglorum*, ed. T. D. Hardy, Eng. Historical Soc. Nos. 6, 7, 1840. Trans. G. A. Giles.

FOR COMPARISON.

	Chaucer's Complete Works, ed. Skeat, Oxford, 1894.
	Guido de Colonna, *Historia Troiana*, Argentina, 1486.
Leahy	Heroic Romances of Ireland, trans. A. H. Leahy, Lon. 1905.
Mabinog.	The Mabinogion, trans. Lady Charlotte Guest. (Quoted by page from Everyman's edition.)
Sec. Sec.	Secreta Secretorum, ed. Robert Steele, EETS. E. S. 74, 1898.

Philos.   Secrees of Old Philosoffres, by Lydgate and Burgh, ed.
                 R. Steele, EETS. E. S. 66, 1894.

RELATED MATERIAL.

BILLINGS, A. H., *A Guide to the Middle English Metrical Romances*, Yale
Studies in English, IX, 1901.

BLÜMMNER, H., *Die Farbenbezeichnungen bei den römischen Dichtern*,
Berl. Stud. f. class. Philol. B 13, H 9.

BUCKHARDT, J., *Die Kultur der Renaissance in Italien*, Leip. 1908.

CLAVIÈRE, R. DE MOULDE DE LA, *Les Femmes de la Renaissance*, Paris, 1904.

FAIRHOLT, F. W., *Costume in England*, Lon. 1896.

GAUTIER, LEON, *La Chivalerie*, Paris, 1895.

GEISSLER, O., *Religion und Aberglaube in den mitteleng. Versromanzen*,
Halle, 1908.

HILL, G., *A History of English Dress*, Lon. 1893.

HOUDOY, J., *La Beaute des Femmes*, Paris, 1876.

JAMES, M., *The Ideal of Personal Beauty in Gower's Confessio Amantis*.
Stanford M. A. Thesis, 1912. (This material is used without further acknowledgment).

LOUBIER, JEAN, *Das Ideal der Maennlichen Schoenheit bei den altfran.
Dichtern des XII und XIII Jahrhunderts*, Halle Diss. 1890.

Mead A.   Mead, Wm. E., *Color in Old English Poetry*, in *Pub.
                 Mod. Lang. Asso.* Vol. XIV. 1899.

Mead B.   Mead, Wm. E., *Color in the English and Scottist Popu-
                 lar Ballads*, in *Furnivall Miscellany*, p. 320 ff.

Ogle I.   Ogle, M. B., Classical Origin of Literary Conceits in
                 English Literature, in *Mod. Lang. Notes*, Vol.
                 XXVII. Dec. 1912; Ogle II. *ibid*, in *Amer. Jour. of
                 Philol.* Vol. XXXIV. 1913; Ogle III. *ibid.* in *The
                 Sewanee Review*, Oct. 1912. (Cf. Further Notes
                 on Classical Literary Tradition, in *Mod. Lang.
                 Notes*, Vol. XXIX, 1914.)

OTT, ANDRÉ, G., *Étude sur les Colours en vieux Français*, Zurich Diss.
Paris, 1899.

SCHULTZ, ALWIN, *Das Höfische Leben zur Zeit der Minnisinger*, Leip. 1889.

SIEFFERT, FRITZ, *Ein Namenbuch zu den altfr. Artusepen*, Greifswald, 1882.

STRUTT, JOS., *Dress and Habits of the People of England*, Lon. 1842.

VOIGT, O., *Das Ideal der Schönheit und Hässlichkeit in den altfranz.
Chansons de Geste*, Marb. Diss., 1891.

WACKERNAGEL, W., *Die Farben- und Blumensprache des Mittelalters*, Leip.
1872. in *Kleinere Schriften*, Vol. I.

Wein AL.   Weinhold, K., *Altnordisches Leben*, Berl. 1856.

Wein DF.   Weinhold, K., *Die Deutschen Frauen in dem Mittel-
                 alter*, 2nd. Edition, Wien, 1882.

WILLMS, JOHANNES EDWARD, *Ueber den Gebrauch der Farbenbezeichnungen
in der Peosie Altenglands*, Münster, 1902.

WRIGHT, THOS., *Womankind in Western Europe*, Lon. 1896.

WOHLGEMUTH, F., *Riesen und Zwerge in den altfranz. erzählenden Dichtung*,
    Tübingen, 1906.

REFERENCE WORKS.

The Century Dictionary.

The Oxford Dictionary, MURRAY-BRADLEY.

HALLIWELL, J. O., *A Dictionary of Archaic and Provincial Words*, Lon. 1847.

JAMIESON, JOHN, *A Scottish Dictionary*, 1882.

BOSWORTH-TOLLER, *Anglo-Saxon Dictionary*, Oxford, 1882.

STRATMANN-BRADLEY, *A Middle English Dictionary*, Oxford, 1891.

INTRODUCTION

Upon a subject so obviously needing treatment as The Middle English Ideal of Personal Beauty very little of a thoro and definite character has as yet been done. Thomas Wright, in his *Womankind in Western Europe,* London, 1879, devotes a few pages (pp. 238 ff.) to the discussion of the type of feminine beauty appreciated in the Middle Ages; but his material is taken, for the most part, from Old French rather than from English sources. *Color in Old English Poetry* by William E. Mead (Cf. Bibl.), and an excellent dissertation, *Ueber den Gebrauch der Farbenbezeichnungen in der Poesie Altenglands,* 1902, by J. E. Willms cover the field of English literature up to the beginning of the fifteenth century. Tho this material is presented from the standpoint of its bearing upon the use of color, still there is much of it which may be used to advantage in reconstructing an ideal of personal beauty. Another dissertation, *Religion und Aberglaube in den mittelenglischen Versromanzen,* Halle, 1908, by O. Geissler devotes one section (p. 54 ff.) to the personal appearance of giants, dwarfs, and dragons. And, finally, there appears a series of recent articles by Professor M. B. Ogle on *The Origin and Tradition of Literary Conceits* (Cf. Bibl.) which are rich in quotations from sixteenth century literature, but which touch but lightly on the field of Middle English literature. These works, together with many scattered notes to individual passages dealing with personal description in the romances especially, comprise, so far as I have been able to ascertain, all that has been done on the subject up to this time.

In a study such as the present one purports to be it is manifestly impossible to cover the entire field of Middle English literature. But to cover any particular period thoroly, or to investigate the entire works of any one school, as for example the Chaucerian, would furnish only a partial and fragmentary

1

view of the subject under discussion. Consequently, as the title
of the work suggests, certain classes of literature have been
selected from which it is possible, I think, to construct a fairly
complete picture of the M.E. ideal of beauty. The results
herein presented are based, primarily, upon an investigation of
the Arthurian, Carlovingian, and Alexandrian cycles of metrical romances, together with other Matter-of-England, Greek,
and Roman romances-of-adventure up to the beginning of the
sixteenth century. Tho personal description is cultivated most
zealously in the romances, it is also found in other classes of
literature as well. Accordingly, legendary material has been
included from the time of *Seinte Marherete* (*ca.* 1200) to
Osbern Bockenam (*ca.* 1440); comprising chiefly the great
collections of Dr. C. Horstmann. In order that personal beauty
as idealized by the creative poet may be supplemented and, to
some degree, corrected by descriptions of more or less historical
personages, all the Chronicles of England have been investi-
gated from Laʒamon's *Brut* to Higden-Trevisa's *Polychronicon*.
Since the chronicles written in English are composed almost
entirely of material drawn from earlier Latin chronicles, a few
of the most important of these have also been included (Cf.
Bibl.). Side-lights are thrown upon the picture thus obtained
by reference to small collections of lyrics from the fourteenth
century. For purposes of comparison, material has been introduced into the notes from Welsh and Old Irish literature, and
from the works of other M.E. writers such as Chaucer and
Lydgate. Undoubtedly the physiognomies must have played a
great part in determining the ideal of beauty in the Middle
Ages, but since the tracing of such an influence lies outside the
scope of this work, I have contented myself with comparative
references to the English translations to which I have had
access. If comparative material is sometimes presented in the
body of the work, it is to throw light upon points not otherwise
sufficiently clear, or to elucidate a rare or obscure word. In the
footnotes have also been placed a great number of observations
gleaned here and there, bearing upon the immediate subject
under discussion.

In the light of the material collected from this field, it appears that the type of beauty appreciated in M.E. literature does not greatly differ from that found in other literatures of medieval times. The descriptions are largely of a set and formal character, and so stereotyped and conventional that we may almost say that there is no distinctively English ideal of beauty. However, the type of feminine beauty praised by the poets in their catalogs of charms is, without an exception, a blonde, whose hair is golden or like gold wire, eyes sparkling bright and light blue in color, cheeks lily-white or rose-red, forehead broad and without wrinkles, red lips, white evenly set teeth, long snow-white arms, and white hands with long slender fingers. Her figure is small, well rounded, slender and graceful, with a small willowy waist as a prime standard of excellence. The skin is everywhere of dazzling whiteness, rivaling the finest silk in softness; and the lower limbs are well formed and as white as milk, with small white and shapely feet. As to the hero of romance and legand, the poet never leaves us in doubt as to his great stature, enormous strength, long sinewy arms, broad square breast and shoulders, together with a small waist and retreating stomach. His legs are long, with thighs thick and strong; and in general appearance he is more like a giant than a mere knight. When his visor is raised, it is seen that his eyes are generally blue in color, with the fierce, proud glance of a falcon; and when his helmet is removed, his golden hair falls down over his shoulders in long curls. It is worthy of note that, tho the golden-haired hero is indeed most highly appreciated, yet he of the long black curling hair holds an almost equal place in the affections of the M.E. poets. Nor is brown or beaverhued hair described except in terms of the highest praise. This broader taste shown in descriptions of men may be due to the influence of the physiognomies, or it may be an appreciation of the Celtic element in the race.[1] At any

---

[1] Cf. *Anglo-Saxon Britain*, Grant Allen, Lon. 1904, p. 56 ff. "We know that the pure Anglo-Saxons were a round-skulled, fair-haired, light-eyed, blonde-complexioned race. . . . But we also know that the Celts, origin-

rate, whatever may be the color of the hair, the warrior's forehead is broad, his features noble and aristocratic. Like that of
a wild animal is his bearing in battle, his voice sounding above
the clamour of the conflict like the roar of a lion or the blast of
a trumpet; but in times of peace he is gentle and mild to
friends, courteous and *debonaire*.

It must not be supposed that all these stereotyped and conventional formulae appear in any one description. Often the
poet deems it sufficient to mention only the lovely golden tresses
of his hero or heroine, the grey eyes and curved eyebrows, the
lady's dazzling white skin and peach-blossom complexion, leaving the filling out of the picture to the reader's imagination.
Such descriptions generally require from one to three lines;

> Alisaunde . . . to-drough his yelow here,   Alis L. 4651.
> With facys white as lely floure,
> With ruddy rede as rose coloure,   Launf. 61.
> Eiȝen gray & browes bent,   Lob. Frau. 34.

While the one-, two-, and three-line descriptions are by far most
common, yet more detailed presentations of beauty are sometimes given. For example, to draw the picture of the fair
Floripas requires eleven lines (Ferum. 5880 ff.), that of Queen
Olympias twenty lines (Alis A. 177 ff.), Hector receives nine-
teen lines (Dest. Tr. 3880.), while Giraldus Cambrensis
devotes thirty-two lines to his description of Eve (*op. cit.* Vol.
I, p. 349.), and the author of the Dest. Troy no less than sixty-
four to the beauty of Helen (Dest. Tr. 3020 ff.).

It may be remarked that, generally, in portrayals of manly
beauty comparatively small space is given to the presentation
of the personal appearance alone. On the other hand, the poet
never tires of heaping up epithets in his attempts to delineate

ally themselves a similar blonde Aryan race, mixed largely in Britain with
one or more long-skulled, dark-haired, black-eyed, brown-complexioned
races, generally identified with the Besques or Eskuarians, and with the
Ligurians. The nation which resulted from this mixture showed traces of
both types, being sometimes blonde, sometimes brunette, sometimes black-
haired, sometimes red-haired, and sometimes yellow-haired." It is with
types of this mixed race that we have to deal in M. E. literature.

the noble and wise character of his hero and to show forth his manly virtues. When Thomas Randolph is introduced by Barbour, no less than twenty-two lines are necessary to enumerate his virtues of prowess, loyalty, and honor (Barb. x. 274 ff.), while three lines must suffice to give some idea of his person;

> He wes of mesurabill stature,
> And portrait weill at all mesure,
> With braid visage, plesand and fair. (Barb. x, 280 ff.)

With this may be compared the ten lines (prose) given to the description of the person of Henry II, and the one hundred-twenty lines required for the delineation of his character (Gir. Camb. v. p. 302 ff.). Tho this tendency to develop character at the expense of personal description is felt most strongly in the chronicles, yet it prevails also to a large extent in the romances as well. That the knight should be " war and wise" (Laȝ. 4174), "moche of myght" (Oct. N. 23.), "stout & stiþe" (Tars. 1092.), "pruddest in palle" (Awn. Arth. 66.), "bold vndur banere" (Avow. Arth. i, 14.), "schene vndir scheild" (Gol. & Gaw. 639.), "stif in stour" (Cur. Mun. 2203.), or noble, courteous, and true is of apparently more importance than that he should be handsome. None are admitted to the fellowship of the Round Table,

> Bot he were noble & douhti kniȝt,
> Strong & hende, hardi & wise,
> Certes & trewe wiþ outen feyntise, Arth. & Merl. 2203.

Probably both the poet and his audience understand that, if the hero is young and of noble birth (as he most always is), valiant, powerful, loyal and true, he is therefore necessarily handsome. The heroine is also often described by means of long series of oft-recurring, more or less colorless epithets. That she is " semely vnþer serke" (Emar. 499.), " godely unþer gore" (*ibid.* 195.), "worthyest in wede" (Torr. 32.), "Luffsum vnder line" (Tris. 2815.), " brihtest vnder bys" (Bödd. W. L. iii. 37.), "markyd vnder mone" (Amad. 616.), or sweet and gentle, meek and mild seems at times to express for the poet her supreme loveliness and exquisite beauty. Still none of these indefinite epithets are given herein except as they appear in definite descriptions of men and women.

No picture of beauty can be considered complete until it is complemented by its opposite, ugliness. It is a peculiarity of the medieval mind to think of beauty as a characteristic of the good, and to look upon ugliness as the distinguishing trait of the evil. Consequently all wicked, malicious, and treacherous persons are presented as being loathsome in their ugliness. The romances abound in descriptions of hideous giants— veritable sons of the Devil—with huge, unshapely bodies, fiery glowing eyes, enormous mouths, bushy eyebrows, black hair, and filthy beards as black as pitch (Cf. Mort. Arth. 1075- 1104.). Dwarfs also appear with their low, deformed bodies, disproportionate limbs and features, broad faces, *camuse* noses, and ugly hair (Cf. Lib. Des. 135 ff.). As may be supposed, the original pattern of all ugliness, the model and prototype of all loathly beings, the Devil, makes frequent appearances in the legends. Doubt not that his face is sooty and black, beard long and unkempt, with hair reaching to his feet; that he has the conventional hooked nose, and that fire is continually flaming from his horrible mouth and eyes (Cf. Sc. Leg. 9. 214.). All enemies of the Christian faith, all unbelievers are, for that very reason, children of the Devil, consequently ugly. It is a common usage in both Legend and Romance to stigmatize all such opponents and enemies with the blasting name, Saracens! If the Saracen, Sir Ferumbras, is pictured as being very hand- some (Ferum. 1822.), it is because he is shortly to be plucked as a brand from the burning, and is destined to become one of the greatest of Christian knights. While, in descriptions of fair persons on the one hand, the poet often suggests their exquisite beauty by a delineation of a wonderfully good and noble character; on the other hand, the utter depravity and wickedness of evil characters is suggested by a detailed descrip- tion of loathly and deformed bodies. Few general epithets are wasted on an ugly giant; to know that he is unutterably evil, it is quite sufficient to describe his repulsive person. If, however, the prime object of the poet is to magnify the prowess of his hero, merely the enormous stature of his opponent is given;.

> Gogmagog was a giant suiþe gret & strong,
> Vor aboute an twenti vet me seiþ he was long, R. Glouc. 508.

Strange to say only a few descriptions of ugly women are to be found; and these are given with the apparent purpose of heightening, thru contrast, the beauty of the heroine (Cf. Gaw. & Gr. Kn. 951 ff.).

Upon the origin of the type of feminine beauty herein described and its perpetuation as a literary tradition in later English literature, the articles by Professor M. B. Ogle offer an able discussion. He shows by means of copious quotations (cf. Ogle III. p. 459.) that the blonde beauty flourishes still in the Elizabethan period as a literary conceit, and that it persists on into modern times. He also shows that " the same type predominates, to the practical exclusion of her dark sister, in the love poetry and prose romances of Italy and France from the 12th century onward; that, moreover, this reign of the blonde in modern literature is but a continuation of her reign in Greece and Rome; that all the Roman love-poets, and the later Greek writers of romance and erotic letters, give to the ladies whom they desire to praise, the same golden or auburn hair, sparkling eyes, white skin, red lips, slender white hands, and that their models, the Greek Alexandrian poets, praise the same blonde type; that, finally, the Greek heroes and heroines, gods and goddesses . . . are described as blondes by Homer and the early poets " (Cf. Ogle II. p. 126.). The prime source not only of the type but also of the literary expression, thinks Professor Ogle, is the literature of the Greek Alexandrian age. " From this drew the Roman Elegiac poets, the writers represented in the Greek Anthology, the professional rhetoricians and the writers of erotic letters and romance; and through them, and especially through the rhetorical schools, the stream passed on into the literature of the entire western world. Beginning with the Renaissance, however, Italian poetry was perhaps the main channel through which traditional conceits were distributed " (Ogle ii. p. 127.).

While in this series of articles no effort is made to trace a direct borrowing from other languages, still by means of a flood of comparative quotations taken from the literatures mentioned, the conclusions stated above seem comparatively well established. In the notes of this study I have introduced copious references to works in Latin, Italian, Old French, Middle High German, and Old Norse dealing with like types of personal beauty, all of which tend to support the theory of Professor Ogle. Reference to these works strongly suggests that not only the entire ideal of both masculine and feminine beauty is borrowed, but also that the ideal of ugliness is taken over in its entirety from other medieval literatures. Moreover, a detailed comparison of Romance and Legend with Old French and Latin sources reveals the unmistakable fact that the very finest and most poetical descriptions in M.E. literature are borrowed. No better example of this could be found than in the Troy stories, where both Lydgate and the author of Dest. Troy are faithful translators of Guide de Colonna, differing only in the matter of phraseology and in their selection of objects of comparison. A comparison of the corresponding passages in certain[2] of the romances and legends with their more or less immediate originals but confirms the statement that, here at least, the general ideal of beauty is borrowed. To make, however, a thoro comparative study of all passages given herein with their immediate sources is not always possible, and even if it were, such a comparison lies outside the range of this work. Detailed comparative passages are given only where there are

---

[2] Compare Ferum. 4435 f. and *Fierabras* 4745 f.; 5879 f. and 2007 f. (cf. 5999.) : 1072 and 1822; Lib. Des. 937 f. and *Bel Inconnu*, 1519 f. (ed. Hippeau) ; Launf. R., 57, 103, 428, and *Lanval*, 61, 105, 569 (ed. Warnke) ; Sc. Leg. ix, 49, 215 and corresponding passages from *Legenda Aurea* (cf. Horstmann, *Legendensammlungen*) ; Alis C. 597 and Latin original in note. A classical example is found in Chaucer's translation of *Le Roman de la Rose* by Jean de Meung and Guillaume de Lorris; and another in Lydgate's *Reson and Sensuallyte*, ed. Sieper, EETS. E. S. 84, 89. Compare ll. 1709-23 with Fr. original in note, also ll. 1569-1600.

striking differences or agreements in phraseology, or where reference to the original throws light on the difficult word.

While most of the poets after the thirteenth century undoubtedly drew upon Latin and Old French models for their descriptions of personal beauty, still there are strong indications to the effect that, originally, the blonde type was independently appreciated by the Anglo-Saxons. Such a conclusion, however, can not be proved, because formal personal description is not known in Anglo-Saxon literature.[3] As F. Roeder remarks in his *Die Familie bei den Angelsachsen,* Halle, 1899, p. 17. "Allein im Gegensatz zu den meisten mittelhochdeutschen Dichtern . . . verzichtet die altenglische Dichtung, die im Schillerschen Sinn 'naiv' ist, auf ausfürliche Schönheitsschilderungen. Sie beschränkt sich darauf, fest geprägte Epitheta, die an sich meist farblos und unplastisch sind, zu wiederholen." Still, as he further notes, a few instances are to be found where light-blonde hair (*hwit-loc, hwit-locced*), with long curls (*wunden-loc*) is highly appreciated among the Anglo-Saxons; and where a white complexion (*blāc hlēor*) is mentioned in terms of the highest praise.[4] In *The Exeter Book Riddles,* ed. Tupper, 1910, at least twice is fair hair given as indicating high rank (Rid. 43, 3; 80, 4.); while dark hair (Rid. 13, 8. *wonfeax Wāle, swearte Wēalas,* 13, 4.) is a distinguishing feature of the Welsh servant class. This attitude of appreciation for the blonde type, and of contempt

[3] (The first detailed description occurs in Cur. Mun. 18830.) Nor can we come to any definite conclusions from a study of the MS. paintings of the Saxons. Strutt is correct when he says, "The figures frequently appear with blue hair; in some instances, which indeed are not so common, the hair is represented of a bright red color; and in others it is of a green and orange hue." But his conclusion that these colors are meant to be realistic is surely far-fetched. He remarks, "I have no doubt in my own mind that arts of some kind were practised at this time to color the hair." Vol. I, p. 73.

[4] Cf. further Bos. Toll. and Grein, *Sprachschatz,* and especially Tupper's notes to *The Exeter Riddles,* 41, 98; 43, 3; 80, 4; 53, 6; 13, 4. I am greatly indebted to Professor Tupper for most of the references contained in this paragraph.

for dark-haired, brown-complexioned races is common in all German antiquity;[5] and I see no reason why an Anglo-Saxon poet, coming from a flaxen-haired, blue-eyed race, should not praise independently a perfect type of that race. Undoubtedly, the Middle English ideal of beauty must have been influenced to some extent by the inherited Anglo-Saxon tradition which happened to coincide with the classical tradition.

Be that as it may, at about the year 1400 the pleasure derived by Middle English poets from the reproductions of long catalogs of personal charms begins to wane. There is felt a tendency skip the pictures and hurry on with the story. For example, the author of *The Laud Troy Book* (ed. Wülfing, EETS. 121-122) leaves out the entire gallery of portraits of the Greek and Trojan heroes, over which Dares, Benôit de Saint More, Guido, the author of Dest. Troy, and Lydgate have spent so much time. He indeed mentions the fact that Dares describes them, but the whole matter is dismissed with two lines,

> Gret tariyng it is to telle
> That Dares makes vpon his spelle.   (Cf. ll. 3317 f.)

Likewise, near the end of the century this tendency is felt—but more strongly. When the author of Partonope of Blois introduces his heroine, he seems very impatient over the long account of her dress found in the French original! He passes over the useless description,

> For eche man wotte well wythowten les,
> A lady þat ys of hye Degree,
> A-rayde in þe beste maner mote be.   Parton. 6178.

He is still more exasperated when he strikes the long list of her charms which he is supposed to translate;

> Whatte nedes to speke of hur forehedde,
> Off hur nose, hur mowþe, hyrre lyppes redde,
> Off hur shappe, or hur armes smalle?
> Off þys and more a ryghte grette tale
> Myne auctor makethe, wych shall not for me

---

[5] Cf. Weinhold, AL. p. 182; Gummere, *Germanic Origins*, p. 59.

> Be nowe rehersed, but thus that she
> Was holden one off the ffayreste
> That was on lyue, and þer-to þe goodelyste
> Wyth to dele þat myghte be,   Parton. 6178 ff.

After this manner are the definite descriptions of the fourteenth century replaced by the indefinite combinations of words in the fifteenth century. It seems quite sufficient to say that the beautiful lady is indescribable or peerless, that she is the fairest alive, or the seemliest creature imaginable, or to refer the gentle reader to the original for a list of her charms.

It may be further suggested that in the time of the Renascence, when foreign literatures were eagerly read and as eagerly translated, when imitations of Latin, Greek, French, and Italian models were made with enthusiasm, the art of cataloging personal charms was again ardently cultivated. The amorous sonnets especially abound in descriptions of personal beauty, the type of which, according to Professor Ogle, is but the continuation of the classical tradition transmitted thru French and Italian channels. But that the prevailing fashion was not universally considered in good taste, is suggested by the fact that in 1575 George Gascoigne, in his *Notes of Instruction,* one of the first works on literary criticism, says;

" If I should vndertake to wryte in prayse of a gentlewoman, I would neither praise hir christal eye, nor hir cherrie lippe, etc. For these things are *trita et obuia.*"

§ 1. HAIR

Practically every detailed description of beauty or ugliness in Middle English literature depends largely for its effects upon the color, length, and condition of the hair. Often the poet gives only this one item in his list of charms, leaving the other characteristics to be inferred. Such an inference is easy enough since, as we have seen, such descriptions more often deal with certain definite and fixed literary types than with the beauty of real personages.

The type of hair most highly appreciated, whether in the descriptions of men or women, youths or maidens, is what we would probably call the blonde.[1] Though the word blonde occurs only once,

þe VI ledde Beliche þe blounde,[2]   (Arth. & Merl. 8707.),

still the term yellow [3] seems to express at different times ideas of all the shades of color from a bright flaxen or yellow to a decided red. When the valiant Guy disguises himself,

His here þat was ȝalu and briȝt,
Blac it become anon riȝt. (Guy A. 6107; B. 5788.) [4]

---

[1] The same is true in the Greek Epic, cf. W. Jordan, *Die Farben bei Homeros*, p. 162 ff. (in Neue Jahrb. für Philol. 1876); also E. Veckenstedt, *Geschichte der greich. Farbenlehre*, p. 136 ff.; and Blümmner, *op. cit.*, p. 106. The Roman poets also express a fondness for blonde hair, probably because it was of rare occurrence, cf. Blümmner, *op. cit.* p. 106 f. In the Old French *only* blonde hair is considered beautiful, cf. Loubier, *op. cit.* p. 44. Voigt, *op. cit.* p. 56, says, "Der bekannte Geschmack der Römer an dem hoch-blonden germanischen Haar hat sich auf das Mittelalter ver-erbt und besonders in Frankreich festen Fuss gefasst." Cf. Gautier, *op. cit.* pp. 205, 374. Houdoy, *op. cit*, p. 36, gives as the reason for this great love of blonde hair, "le blonde était le signe distinctif de la race pure, une sorte d'attribut national, auquel on attachait un grand prix." Sieffert, on the other hand, finds, "Man kan . . . schliessen, dass schwarzes Haar bei den Franzosen das Normal ist . . . dass das Seltene in hohen Ansehen steht," *op. cit.* p. 16. In Old French the particular shade of yellow desired is a " jaune éblouissant, jaune vif," Ott, *op. cit.* p. 87. Likewise in the Middle High German only the gold-blonde is praised, cf. Schultz, *op. cit.* I. 212; Wackernagel, *op. cit.* p. 190; Weinhold DF. p. 223. In Old Norse blonde or yellow is at least the most highly prized color for hair, cf. Weinhold AL. p. 21; *Archœl.* XXIV. p. 253. For certain Italian writers of the Renaissance with like ideals of beauty, cf. Buckhardt, *op. cit.* II. p. 65; Clavière, *op. cit.* p. 272. For peoples of Western Europe, including the English, cf. Wright, *op. cit.* p. 238. For other citations in Middle English, cf. Willms, *op. cit.* pp. 65-67; and for later quotations and other references to sources, cf. Ogle I. p. 237; II. p. 127 f.; III. 462; Mead B. p. 331.

[2] Ital. *biondo* (cf. Buckhardt, *op. cit.* p. 65, vol. II.); Med. Lat. *blondus*, *blundus*, yellow (DuCange, *flavus qui vulgo dicitur blondus.*). Related to A.S. *beblonden*, dyed, and *blonden*, to mix (cf. Bos-Toll.). "Hence DuCange conjectures the original sense to be ' dyed,' the ancient Germans being accustomed to dye their hair yellow." Cit. from Murray.

[3] Cf. Skeat's Chaucer, vol. v. p. 65.

[4] See further for beautiful yellow hair Arth. & Merl. 858; Sev. Sag. 477;

Likewise in Laȝamon 18448 is found once " falewe [5] lockes," which Madden translates " yellow locks." The Latin chronicles use the term *flavus* [6] to express the desired color of blonde hair. Of Eve it is said,

> *Perque humeros flavas projicit illa comas,* Gir. Cam. I. 352.

Yellow as gold [7] is a common comparison used to intensify the charm of the color as well as to give some idea of the lustre of beautiful hair. Of the fair flower-women, who grow up in the spring and die down again in the autumn, the poet says,

> Heore heir heore clothyng ys,
> Al so yalow so any gold. Alis L. 6494 f. (Cf. *ibid.* 4989.)

The handsome Paris has,

> Here huet on his hede as haspis of silke,
> And in sighkyng it shone as the shyre golde, Dest. Tr. 3899.

(Comp. Lyd. II. 4902, and Guido, *flavus coma, quod eius tota cesaries nitorem aureum presentaret,* sig. e₂verso₂).

Yellow as wax [8] is a comparison occasionally found applied

Alis L. 207, 1999, 4651; Ferum. 5881; Horst B. Misc. 3. 95; Horst C. p. 493; Horst D. 59. 182; 66. 96; Hig-Trev. VIII. 63; Dest. Tr. 3968 and Lyd. II. 4956, comp. Guido, *crinibus autem crispatis et flauis,* Memnon. sig. e₂ verso₂); Kn. of Cour. 178, 212, 382, 440; Gower VII. 4881.

[5] A.S. *fealo,* " pale yellow, shading into red or brown." Mead A. p. 198.

[6] *Flavus,* golden yellow inclining to red, cf. Blümner, *op. cit.* p. 105. The description in Gir. Cam. v. 323, *capillis flavis et subscripsis,* is translated by the author of Conq. Ire. p. 98, " yolowe her & sam-crysp." Cf. further Gir. Cam. VIII. 127; IV. 47; Wm. Malms. 213, 504.

[7] Comp. the Old Irish " And their hair . . . shone golden their shoulders round," Leahy II. p. 11; " hair gold-yellow " *ib.* p. 151; " the top of the head of primrose," *ib.* p. 155; " hair yellow and fair," *ib.* I. p. 8. For the Welsh cf. Mabinog. p. 183, " And the man had two sons, the one had yellow hair, and the other had auburn." Chaucer satirizes the conceit, *Can. Tales,* B, 1920.

> His heer, his berd was lyke saffroun.

For beautiful yellow hair—*val* or *gel*—compared to gold in the German, cf. Wackernagel, *op. cit.* p. 164. Comp. Ogle I. p. 237; II. p. 128 f.; III. 462; and Tupper, F. *op. cit.* pp. 95, 170.

[8] The same comparison, expressing beauty, is found in the German, cf. Wackernagel, *op. cit.* p. 165. Cf. also Kaluza in note to Lib. Des. 139, and Kölbing in *Engl. Stud.* XI. 499.

to the hair, but more often to the beard. (Cf. § 2.). Chaucer's Pardoner is a classic example,

> This pardoner hadde heer as yelow as wex.
> But smothe it heng as dooth a strike of flax.   C. Tales, A. 675 f.

If Willms remarks (*op. cit.* p. 67.) that this comparison is " niemals auf das Haupthaar mit dem Nebengriff der Schönheit angewandt," he is generalizing too hastily from the single quotation given above. As a matter of fact the Pardoner's hair is not ugly because it is as yellow as wax, but because it hangs straight and smooth. Willms is also evidently unacquainted with the following quotation,

> Then they lowsyd hur feyre faxe,
>   That was yelowe as the waxe,
> And schone also as golde redd.   (Bon. Flor. 1545.)

and with a charming description of Ajax in the *Laud Troy Book,*

> A louely knyght that het Ayax,
> With lokkis faire, ȝelow as wax,
> Hongyng side aboute his swyre.   l. 15615.

Kaluza (Lib. Des. CLIV.) further quotes from a description of a dwarf found in *Sir Degarre,* ed. Miller, Edin. 1849;

> Bothe his berd and his fax
> Was crisp and ȝhalew as wax.   l. 783 f.

Yellow as glass occurs once, used in the description of probably the same dwarf mentioned above;

> the hayre that on his head was,
> looked as yellowe as any glasse.   Degree P. 647 f.

Gold. Many are the passages where lovely hair is said to be like gold [9] both in color and in lustre. The famous description

---

[9] Comp. the Old Irish, " a lady, Like gold is her hair," Leahy I. p. 73; " Curling golden hair, Fair as gems it shone," *ibid.* 148; " Golden-haired with long tresses," *ibid.* 92; " On her head were two tresses of golden hair, and each tress had been plaited into four strands, at the end of each strand was a little ball of gold," *ibid.* p. 13. For later English literature, cf. William Heise, *Die Gleichnisse in Edmund Spenser's Faerie Queene,* Strass.' Diss. 1902, p. 38. Curiously enough an early description of the

of Eve begins with the words, *Aurea cesaries* (Gir. Cam. I. 349), and her fairest daughter, Helen, is presented,

> The here of hir hede, huyt as the gold,
> Bost out vppon brede bryght on to loke,   Dest. Tr. 3021.

(Guido, *Miratur . . . in ea rutilanti flauescere crines multos*, sig. d₃ ver. 2.). Compare further " Lemond as gold," Dest. Tr. 459; " flammet of gold," *ib.* 4135 (cf. Lyd. II. 4984); " colouret as gold," *ibid.* 3757; " Ech her semede of gold," Ferum. 5881; " hare schenand as gold scho hade," Sc. Leg. 34, 19 (not in *Leg. Aurea, corpore pulcherrima*); " all of fresh gold shone her heade," Eger & Gr. 216, 794.   In this last quotation the gold may refer to the head-dress, but I am inclined to think the poet means to compare the hair to " fresh gold."

Gilt.   Exceedingly rare are descriptions of gilt hair.   Of Andromache it is said,

> Gilde hores hade þat gay, godely to se,   Dest. Tr. 3989.

(Comp. Lyd. II. 4985, Lik gold hir tresses; and Guido, *cesarie de aurata*, sig. e₃ recto 1.).   Chaucer [10] has the only other example which I have been able to find,

> Hyd, Absolon, thy gilte tresses clere.   Leg. Good Wom. 249.

Auburn.   There is one occurrence of auburn hair; namely, in Lydgate's description of the handsome Achilles,

> With hawborne her, crisping for þikness.   Lyd. II. 4550.

Here the word auburn has its original meaning [11] of bright or

Devil says " his lockes ant his longe berd blikede al ogolde," Marh. fol. 43. This is not to be taken as the real color of the hair, however; the monster has just been gilded over—hence the description.

[10] Chaucer has also the comparison, like burned gold, which I have not found elsewhere, " Hir heer . . . As burned gold his shoon to see," H. Fame, 1386 f.

[11] In O. Fr. " Auburn et aubornez créent une nouvelle maniere d'exprimer, jaune dans le sens de ' blanchatre,' ' blanc jaune,' ' jaune brilliant.' " Ott, *op. cit.* p. 87.   In M. E. it has the meaning of citron-colored (cf. Promptorum Parv. *citrinus*), or whitish, flaxen-colored (cf. DuCange, *alburnus, subalbus*).   The modern meaning of chestnut-brown came in about the sixteenth century, probably as the result of the accent of the last syllable —abrûn.   Cf. Murray, Century, Loubier, *op. cit.* p. 47.

light yellow, since it translates Guido's description, *flauis crinibus sed crispatis,* sig. e₁ verso 2. (Comp. Benoit, Crespes chevus
ot e aubornes, *Roman de Tr.* 5161; and Dares, *capillo myrteo,*
cap. XII.)

Gold Wire. A favorite object of comparison with Middle
English poets is gold wire.[12] Beautiful hair shines like gold
wire, or is as yellow as gold wire, or as bright and glistening.

> Seoððen com a king hæhte Pir,
> His hæð (read head) wes swulc beoð gold wir.   Laȝ. 7047.

This seems to be original with Laȝamon since the corresponding
passage in Wace runs,

> Pir qui ot le cief mult bel,   3800.

See further,

> Her her was to her Knees as red as gold wyre,   Wed. Gaw. 744.
> Hir hed was ȝolow as wyre
> Of gold fyned wiþ fyre,   Pist. Sus. 192 f.
> Here here shynyng on her hede
> As gold wyre yn somer bright,   Launf. R. 433.

(Cf. Launf. M. 938, and compare Lanval, ed. Warnke, fils d'or
ne gete tel luur cum si chevel cuntre le jur, 575 f.).
The description,

> With her long as gold wire on the grene (Bev. M. 400),

has absolutely no basis in the French original (cf. *Boeve de
Hamtone,* 373 f. ed. Stimming); but the following,

> þe her schon on hir heed,
> As gold wire schineþ briȝt (Lib. Des. 938)

is evidently an attempted translation of *Le Bel Inconnu* (ed.
Hippeau),

> Les crins ot blons et reluisans,
> Comme fin or reflanboians, l. 1529 f.

(Cf. Troy H. 641; Lyd. II. 4902, 4743; IV. 590; Alis. A. 180;
Parton. Fragm. 41.). The comparison, like gold wire, is proba-

---

[12] For other citations cf. Kölbing to Bev. M. 400; Heise, *op. cit.* 38;
Schick to Lyd's. Temple of Glass, 271; comp. Mead B. p. 332; Ogle, III.
463.

bly the outgrowth of the custom of attiring the hair with gold
wire or threads. Of Queen Olympias it is said,

> Hire yolowe heir was faire atyred,
> With riche strynges of gold wyred, (Alis. L. 207; comp. Lyd. II. 4741),

and Wm. Malmsbury describes the head-dress of Athelstan with
capillo flavo filis auries pulchre intorto, p. 213. Still it may be
but the English way of translating the similar comparison, like
gold threads, which is so common in other literatures.[13]

Red as Gold is also sometimes applied to beautiful hair;

> The comlly heare as golde so rede,   Kn. of Cour. 343;
> Her her was to her knees as red as gold wyre,   Wed. Gaw. 744.

(Cf. Bon. Flor. 1545.). Mead A. (p. 195.), remarking on the
convention of calling gold red, says that it "may be due to the
fact that the gold of that time was often darker than that of our
own, and contained a considerable alloy of copper." Hair red
as gold, then, would be dark gold-blonde, inclining to brown.

Sunbeam. The lustre of golden hair is often compared to the
brightness of the sunbeam,

> Hire hed when ich beholde apon,
> þe sonnebeem aboute noon me þohte þat y-seʒe,   Bödd. W. L. v. 13.

A very poetical passage describes the beauty of Polyxena, rend-
ing her hair in grief,

> When the hond of that hend to þe hede yode,
> Hit semyt by sight of sitters aboute,
> As the moron mylde meltid aboue,
> When he hasted with hond þe hore for to touche,   Dest. Tr. 9139.

It is a conceit beloved especially by Lydgate to compare bright
sunny hair to the beams of Phoebus in his sphere,

> Hir golden her, lik þe schene stremys
> Of fresche Phoebus with his briʒte bemys,   Lyd. II. 3663.

---

[13] Cf. Schultz, *op. cit.* I. 212; Weinhold D. I. 224; and *Archæl.* XXIV. 253,
"Harfagar, who ascended the throne of Norway about A. D. 866, derived
his name from the length and beauty of his hair which is said to have
flown down in thick ringlets to his girdle, and to have been *like golden
or silken threads.*"

2

(Cf. further Lyd. ii. 4741; iv. 590; Lyd's *Temple of Glass,* 1. 271 and Schick's note to same for many other citations.)

Red. Only a few times is red hair mentioned directly, and these are found in workings over of the Troy stories. The King of Persia of course has a fiery head of hair,

> The here of þat hathell was huet as þe fire,
> Bothe o berde & aboue all of bright rede,   Dest. Tr. 3857,

(comp. Lyd. ii. 4769; Guido, *capillos et barbam velut igneam rubicundam,* sig. e₂ recto 2); and Menelaus likewise is described,

> His hed was red his berd also,   Troy B. 805.

(Comp. Troy H. 697; Dares, *rufum,* cap. xii; Jos. of Exeter, *comae geniale rubentes.*) Of the somewhat deformed and ugly Frederick I, the description runs, *crines rutile, barba rubens, utrimque interfusa canities (erant),* Gir. Cam. viii. 279. Blümmner remarks apropos of the adjective *rutilus,* " dass dieselbe auch mit dem Blond nahe verwandt ist; es ist offenbar jenes gold-rothe Haar gemeint, das sich durch seinen wunderbaren metallischen Glanz auszeichnet." *op. cit.* p. 179.

As to the term, " the red," which is given often as a kind of nickname to certain characters, Willms (*op. cit.* p. 45.) supposes that it has reference to the color of the hair. Undoubtedly so; but it may also be descriptive of the face, respectively the beard or, which is most probable, it may refer to the general impression of redness given by hair, beard, and face. " William þe rede king " (R. Glouc. 7621, 7607, 7827, 7853, 8022, 8560, 9641) is later described as being,

> þoru out red mid grete wombe,   (*ibid.* 8571.),

which is an attempted translation of Wm. Malms., with *colore rufo, crine subflavo,* (p. 504. Cf. further Hav. 1396; Arth. & Merl. 5443, 5484.) Whether red hair is to be considered ugly or not, cannot be determined,[14] but in connection with red skin

---

[14] In the Latin (*rufus*) is considered exceedingly ugly, cf. Blümmner, 176. Also in Old French, " L'ancien Francais semble avoir tenu en grande aversion la chevelure et la peau rousses, cette coleur lui déplaisant, roux devint

and beard it is to be held in suspicion.[15] As the physiognomist remarks, " Tho that bene rede men, bene Parceuynge and trechurus, and full of queyntise, i-likenyd to Foxis." (Sec. Sec. 229), and later, speaking of the hair, says, " Reede coloure tokenyth a man angri and vicious," Sec. Sec. 233. As far back as the time of King Alfred this same distrust of the red man is felt and expressed;.

> þe rede mon he is a quede
> for he wole þe þin iwil rede,
> he is a cocher, þef and horeling,
> Scolde, of wrechedome is king. Prov. of Alfred, 702 f. Cf. 678 f.

It is worthy of note, however, that in the Old Irish and Welsh [16] red hair seems to be appreciated, tho to a less extent than the blonde.

Brown. The descriptive adjective brown [17] when applied to hair may mean any shade varying thru indefinite degrees from a decided chestnut-brown to black.[18] This color of hair seems to have been of greatest appeal to Middle English poets—next after the blonde—and especially to the clerics, who probably knew of the physiognomist's observation, " Broune lockys and a-broune tokenyth loue of ryght and Justice," Sec. Sec. 233.

sunonyme de laid." Ott, *op. cit.* 107, cf. Loubier, *op. cit.* 48. Among the north Germans red hair is not considered ugly, since it is the distinctive sign of the class of freedman, Weinhold AL. 181. If the hair is not the desired colour, it is dyed red, cf. Wackernagel, *op. cit.* 190.

[15] So in the German, cf. Wackernagel, *op. cit.* p. 172 f. As to the source of the aversion, he thinks it originated among the German people, and is probably connected with the fable of Odysseus, the Fox. His first quotation is from the year 1000, p. 177. The epithet, the red, carries with it no idea of reproach, cf. *ibid.* p. 174. Comp. Sec. Sec. 114; Philos. 2579 f.

[16] Cf. Mabinog. pp. 187, 196. Cf. also The Wooing of Emer (*Archæl. Rev.* I.) translated from the Celtic by Kuno Meyer, where the red hair of the heroine seems to have deeply impressed the poet. Cit. from H. Ellis, The Colour Sense in Literature, *Contemp. Rev.* LXIX, p. 715 f.

[17] Found only a few times in Old French, cf. Loubier, *op. cit.* p. 48. Chestnut-brown is favored in certain northern countries, cf. Weinhold AL. p. 181. Comp. appreciative description of auburn hair in Mabinog. p. 176, 191, 196, 206, 185.

[18] Wackernagel supposes *brûn* to mean black in M. H. German, in O. Norse and in certain *märchen* which he cites, p. 165.

The author of Cur. Mundi lingers apparently with peculiar pleasure over the detailed description of the nut-brown hair of the Christ;

> His heer like to þe note broun,
> Whenne hit for ripe falleþ doun,
> Vpon his shuldres liggyng well,
> Bi his eres slydynge som dell, l. 18833 ff.

Saint Marguerite follows the Christ with

> lockes þat ben broun, (Horst. C. Misc. 3. 344.),

and of St. Bartholomew likewise it is said,

> his her is broun and swiþe crips, Horst. D. 55. 64.

In this latter passage " broun" is probably an indefinite dark color approaching black since St. Bartholomew is described in the *Leg. Aurea* with *capilli . . . crispi et nigri* (cf. Horst. *Legendensammlungen,* 9. 49.), and is presented with black hair in all the other legends. On this same order is the hair of Henry I. He has " brune here" in R. Glouc. (8841), which is a translation of Wm. Malms., with *crine nigro,* p. 642. In the description of a beautiful knight, Salome, the poet, being impressed by the dark shade of his hair, says,

> His hed was crolle and yolow the here,
> Broune thereonne, and white his swere, Alis. L. 1999 f.

To intensify the impression of the whiteness of the hair of one of the seven wise men, it is said,

> His hare was white and nathing brown, (Sev. Sag. 79 f.);

and to avoid any possible misunderstanding, of the fairest we are told,

> His haire was blayke and nothing brown, *ibid.* 117.

In connection with Arthur's noble knights occurs the single reference to beaver-colored hair,

> Alle bare heuede . . . with beveryne [19] lokkes, Mort. Arth. 3631.

---

[19] Cf. Murray, " reddish-brown"; Mätzner, " biberfarbig, broun, ins Röt-liche oder Gelbliche fallend."

Of a strange people, whose hair changes color every ten years, is it said,

> Of nynetene wyntres and an half
> Hy ben hore also a wolf,
> And when hy ben thritty yaar,
> Hy ben broun of hare as hy weren aar,
> And so ay, by the ten yere,
> The coloure chaunges of her here,   Alis. L. 5030 f.

In many cases we find merely the epithet "the brown," [20] which, as Willms supposes (*op. cit.* p. 57.), has reference to the color of the hair. I am of the opinion that it may also at times refer to the color of the skin and face as well.

> þe xvi was Amores þe broun,   Arth. & Merl. 5441.

(Cf. further *ibid.* 5631, 5636, 9069; Horst. C. 234, 344; Horst. C. Misc. p. 193, 19; Havel. 1008, 1909, 1945, 2181, 2249, 2694, 2847, 1750.). Sometimes, however, the word seems to have lost its original meaning, and to be on a par with other indefinite epithets such as hardy, noble, and good;

> He was mickel, broun and beld,   Arth. & Merl. 1190.

Black. In Middle English literature black hair is considered very beautiful,[21] provided it is nicely curled and otherwise well attended to. In the chronicles we find even bishops, nobles, and kings have black hair. Henry I is described with *crine nigro* (Wm. Malms. 642.), Paulinus with *nigro capillo* (Hen. Hunt. p. 87.), and the Abbot Samson is handsome, *paucos canos habens in rufa barba, paucissimos inter capillos nigros et aliquantulum*

---

[20] In Old French, "Der Name li Bruns, findet sich eigentumlicherweise bei Rittern, die gegen die bestehenden Gesetze verstossen oder sich sonstige Ungehörigkeiten erlauben." Sieffert, *op. cit.* p. 16.

[21] On the contrary, in Old Norse black hair is considered decidedly ugly, cf. Weinhold, *op. cit.* AL. pp. 31, 181. Likewise in O. Fr. cf. Loubier, *op. cit.* 49: Sieffert, *op. cit.* p. 16; Houdoy, *op. cit.* p. 37; also in the Latin, cf. Blümmner, *op. cit.* pp. 43, 56, 95. Among the South Germans black hair is considered ugly or at least foreign, cf. Weinhold DF. I. 224;. comp. Schultz, *op. cit.* I. 220. In the *Rigs Mâl* black hair is a sign of serfdom, cf. Wackernagel, *op. cit.* p. 190. In the physiognomies black hair betokens a man of justice and right dealings, cf. Philos. 2552, 2577; Sec. Sec. p. 114.

crispos.[22]   Joc. Brak. 29.   Barbour, speaking of the Black Douglas (xv, 538), says,

> Bot he wes nocht so fayr, that we
> Suld spek gretly off his beaute. . . .
> In wysage wes he sumdeill gray,
> And had blak har   (I. 381.),

but he hastens to add that,

> Ector had blak har as he had. . . .
> & wes curtais and wyss and wycht.   *ibid.* 397 ff.

The ordinary description of St. Bartholomew says that he is *nigri capilli capitis* (Gir. Cam. II. 68.), or, to quote from the legends,

> His hare is crisp and als cole blac,   Horst. C. 24. 86.

Cf. Sc. Leg. 9. 49 and Cur. Mun. 22510.   In the Troy story Ajax T, the beautiful, is described as being

> Blake horit, aboue breghis and other,
> Serklyt of hom seluyn, semly with all,   Dest. Tr. 3780.

Cf. Lyd. II. 4584 (Guido, *nigris . . . crinibus sed circulatis,* sig. e₁ ver. 2).   Of Neoptholomus it is said,

> His here was hard blake on his hede stode,   Dest. Tr. 3820.

(Cf. Lyd. II. 4645, " blak schynyng as doþ get " and Guido, *crinibus nigris* sig. e₂ recto 1).   It is worthy of note that in the description of Ajax T neither of the translators thinks it worth while to reproduce Guido's qualifying *sed;* in fact one English poet is so far enamoured of black hair that Achilles, who generally has golden hair, is described,

> And his hed was as Mahoun,   Troy B. 1287.

Further, Charlemagne contrary to the customary white-hair description is pictured as being

[22] Comp. the red beard and black hair with those of an ugly dwarf, " the moste contirfet and foulest that eny hadde sein, ffor he was deformed, and his browes reade and longe, and his berde reade and longe, that henge down to his breste, and his heeir was grete and blakke and foule medled." Merlin, ed. Mead, W. E.   EETS. 36, 112, p. 635.

> Blac of here & rede of face,   (Rol. & Vern. 434.) ;

of the sixth Sage, the very fairest of them all, it is said,

> His haire was blayke and nothing broun   (Sev. Sag. 117.) ;

and the exceedingly handsome knight whom Arthur meets is described,

> With bere hedes of blake, browed ful bolde   (Awn. Arth. 385.).

I have found only three passages where the idea of ugliness is associated directly with black hair. After Guy has disguised himself, we learn,

> His here þat was ʒalu and briʒt,
> Blac it become anon riʒt   (Guy. A. 6107),

and Orpheus after a long wandering in search of Eurydice is described,

> The here of his hede is blak and row,
> Benethe his gurdel it ys ygrow.   Orph. 253.

In this latter quotation the idea of ugliness seems to be attached, not so much to the blackness of the hair, as to its roughness and its being long and unkempt. Finally, of a hideous giant it is said,

> Hys hed is row wyth feltred here,
> Blake brysteld as a bore.   Ipom. 6147. (Comp. Alis. L. 6260 f.)

Here too the ugliness is largely found in the idea of the hair's being coarse as a boar's bristles, and matted with filth. However, since almost all ugly giants, dwarfs, and Saracens have black beards, or black hides, or are rough like certain animals it may reasonably be supposed that they also have black hair.[23]

Strangely enough, black hair is not mentioned at all in connection with feminine beauty [24] or ugliness. In the Celtic, it may be remarked, both men and women with long, well-attired, glossy black hair are considered beautiful.[25] I should like to

---

[23] For characteristics of the traditional giant and dwarf in O. Fr. cf. Wohlgemuth, *op. cit.* pp. 32, 81.

[24] For a discussion of the very few women in all literature with black hair cf. Ogle I. 241, note 63; *ibid.* II. 126, note 1; *ibid.* III. 460.

[25] Cf. Mabinog., " I was looking upon the snow and upon the raven and

suggest that it is probably the fusion of the Celtic with the Teutonic element in the race represented by the Middle English people which is responsible for the high favor shown to the black-haired as well as to the blonde type in Mid. Eng. literature. In Chaucer we find that the King of Inde, whose hair " was yelow and glitered as the sone " (Cant. Tales, A. 2165.), is in no wise preferred in personal beauty to the King of Trace, of whom it is said,

> His longe heer was kembed bihinde his bak,
> As any ravenes fether it shoon for blak. C. T., A. 2143.

Grey hair [26] is found a great number of times, and is generally venerated and respected as the distinctive sign of age. It is described as being hoar, white-hoar, gray-hoar, white, white as wool or as milk or as the driven snow, or gray as a wolf.[27]

> *Hoar.*   þa fond he þer ane quene. . . .
> heor-lockede wif. Laʒ. 25843, 25867.
> With white-hore heued & berd y-blowe,
> As white as ani driuen snowe. Guy A. St. 45. 10.

---

upon the droops of blood of the bird that the hawk had killed upon the snow. And I bethought me that her whiteness was like that of the snow, and that the blackness of her hair and of her eyebrows like that of the raven, and that the two red spots upon her cheeks were like the two drops of blood," p. 194. A similar version is found in the Old Irish where a raven comes down to drink the blood of a calf slain on the snow, then . . . " his hair as black as the raven, his cheeks red like the blood, and his body white as the snow." Leahy, *op. cit.* I. p. 94; cf. also Mabinog. p. 187. For a like story in other languages cf. J. Grimm, *Märchen*, No. 53; *Altd. Wäldren*, I. 10. In the note to *Märchen* 53 Grimm shows that the story in various forms is found in almost every language, which leads Wackernagel (*op. cit.* p. 164.) to suppose that there is no borrowing of any language from another, but that each story has an independent growth. The presence of black in connection with white and red, he says, is only to bring out the beauty of the latter colors by contrast. For the arguments in support of a Celtic origin, however, cf. *The Wife of Bath's Tale*, by J. H. Maynadier, App. C.

[26] For many other quotations from Early and Middle English cf. Willms, *op. cit.* pp. 21, 26, 30, 36; Mead A. pp. 192, 190; comp. *Beowulf*, ll. 608, 1593, 1790, 1872, 2961. Cf. Chaucer, C. T., A. 3870 for " mouldy hairs " and Skeat's note, Vol. v. 113.

[27] Comparisons in M. E. are not so rich as in O. Fr., " white as flower in April, or as fine silver, or as ivory, or snow," cf. Ott, *op. cit.* pp. 9, 35,

Cf. further, An hore y-blowe kniȝt, Guy A. 3835; hore also a
wolf, Alis. L. 5030; hore hed, Ferum. 154, 1580, 3191, 5475;
Arth. & Merl. 2701; Oct. S. 1919; Lib. Des. 703, 972; Max.
75, 125, 264; Trev. I. 81, 83, 365; Horst. D. 36. 265, 618;
39. 145; 47. 237; 61. 62; 66. 330; 74. 56; Guy. C. 85; Pist.
Sus. 58; Gamel. 817; Horst. A. 3. 857, 907; Parton. 7595;
Lanc. 365; Guy B. 4775, 8565, 9671, 11004, 11081, 11803.
The epithet, the hoar, is sometimes found, " Ermyn þe hore,"
Bev. A. 725, 3322, 3968, 4005.   The faded lover laments her
unloveliness in old age,

> For loves lust and lockes hore,
> In chaumbre acorden nevermore.   Gower VIII. 2403, 2831.

An exceedingly ugly hag is described as follows,

> Hir front was nargh, hir lockes hore,
> Sche loketh forth as doth a More.   Gower I. 1685.

It is here worthy of suggestion, it seems to me, that " hore " in
this connection does not mean " hoary " as Macaulay says (cf.
Gloss.), but rather it carries with it the idea of dirty, filthy.[28]
Her locks are so matted, tangled, and unkempt that it is said of
her later,

> Bot with no craft of combes brode,
> Thei myhte hire hore lockes schode,   Gower I. 1750.

White.   Of Rohand, the aged master of Tristan, we are told,

> His heued was white of hare,   Tris. 686.

Cf. further Sev. Sag. 78; Sc. Leg. 18. 225; Guy B. 7408; Bon.
Flor. 87; Trev. I. 144; Grail 15.639; Parton. 2524, 7171,
7972, 9398; Guy B. 11129; " heire white as mylke in coloure,"
Trev. VII. 266; "hire her was hor and swiþe ȝwijȝt as þei it
were wolle," Horst. D. 39. 145.   The term white is not always

---

42. Cf. Blümmner, *op. cit.* pp. 5, 23, 35 for such comparisons in the
Latin.

[28] Related to O.E. *horig*, M.L.G. *horeg*, H.H.G. *horec*, filthy, dirty.   Comp.
O. E. *horu*, dirt, filth, and *horȝen*, to cover with filth, cf. Bos-Toll, Stratt-
Brad.

used to denote age, but may sometimes be used as synonymous with beautiful.   Merlin's mother, who is young and very beautiful, has

White hayre & long arme   (Arth. & Merl. P. 680.),

and a young child which appears in a vision to St. Dorothea has

white loxe crispe and pure.   Horst. B. Misc. 7. 277.

A beautiful god is described as having grey or white hair,

His cheulere as chauele for changing of eld,   Alis. C. 4924.

(Cf. Skeat's note and Latin original, *caput . . . tanquam purissima lana*).   An ugly monster also has grey hair,

A grym grisely gome with grete gray lokis,   Alis. C. 4956.

The word *lyard,* meaning gray,[29] seems to carry with it the idea of ugliness when applied to hair.   I find it only once,

The lokkes lyarde and longe the lenghe of a ȝerde,   Mort. Arth. 3281.

Besides being of a certain hue,[30] beautiful hair must be long, curling or crisp, and well kempt.   The custom of wearing the hair long is of great antiquity, going back to the Gauls, Danes, Saxons, and Britons.   At certain periods in history the custom has been carried to such an excess as to call down upon it the censure of the Church and her unworldly-minded votaries, resulting in its abandonment for long periods at a time.[31]   But in the Middle English period noble men and women wear long

---

[29] Cf. Donaldson, Introd. to Dest. Tr. xxi; Kölbing to Ipom. 3892; Skeat to Chaucer, Vol. v. p. 328.

[30] Tho the custom of dyeing the hair is ancient and prevalent enough at this time (cf. Strutt, *op. cit.* II. p. 126), I find only two references to it in M.E. literature.   The author of Cur. Mundi reproaches the belles of his time,

And studies hu your hare to heu   (Cur. Mun. 28013),

and Partonope, prematurely gray from sorrow, has recourse to an ointment made from a " certeyn asshe," which is said to have improved the color of his hair hugely.   Parton. 7596.

[31] For full history of the custom cf. Strutt, *op. cit.* II. p. 140; Hill, *op. cit.* pp. 6, 13, 21 f.; and especially *Archæl.* xxiv. p. 252 f.

hair,[32] tho there are not wanting fiery preachers against the custom.

Women's hair is sometimes described as being merely long, sometimes as reaching to the waist or to the knees or to the feet, and often it is long and thick enough to serve as clothing for the whole body.

> Hire lockes lefely aren & longe, Bödd. W. L. v. 31.

Cf. Alis. A. 180; Cur. Mun. 13704; Thos. Ercel. 54; Dest. Tr. 9124; Gower, V. 317; Lyd. II. 4741; Horst. D. 69, fol. 199 a[3]; Horst. B. Misc. 2. 145; Large tresses, Guy C. 67. A more definite description of the hair of Queen Olympias says,

> Hire yolowe heir . . . wryen hire aboute al,
> To hire gentil myddel smal. Alis. I. 207.

Not the least striking characteristic of Dame Ragnell become beautiful is that her hair reaches

> to her knees as red as gold wyre (Wed. Gaw. 744),

and another fair woman has hair

> Fulle bloye, wyche hynge downe to hyr fete. Parton. 6161.

Still further it is said of beautiful Flower Women that

> Hoere heir heore clothyng ys [33] (Alis. L. 6494),

and Trev. does not fail to give the famous incident of Godiva riding thru the streets with no clothing except her hair. (Trev. VII. 199.). This idea of women's hair being long enough to serve as clothing for the body is found especially in the legends, where female saints are given long hair as a particular mark of

---

[32] Long hair is also appreciated in other countries, cf. Schultz, *op. cit.* I. 286; Weinhold DF. I. 223; Wackernagel, *op. cit.* p. 190; Voigt, *op. cit.* p. 56; Loubier, *op. cit.* 55; Weinhold AL. 180; Trev. I. 354; Buckhardt, *op. cit.* p. 65, vol. II. Cf. Strutt, II. 126, for the custom in Eng. of wearing false hair. For great appreciation of long hair in *The English and Scottish Popular Ballads*, ed. F. J. Child, cf. Index under "hair."

[33] For same conceit in German cf. Weinhold DF. I. p. 223; and in Old Norse cf. Weinhold AL. 182.

grace from God to cover their shame when disrobed for torture.
The poet says of St. Agnes that,

> quhene hire clathis al of ware,
> god send sic sydnes in hyre hare,
> þat scho wes cled mare ewinely
> with hare þane with hire clathes.   Sc. Leg. 41. 157.

(Cf. same account Boc. 6. 325; Horst. D. 29. 48, 72, and compare *Leg. Aurea, Tantam autem densitatem capillis ijus dominus contulit ut melius capillis quam vestibus tegeretur,* Horst. *Legendensammlungen,* 41. 157. Comp. Sc. Leg. 50. 978; Horst. C. 18. 226.). On the other hand, St. Egipciane, who has held to the wilderness for many years and is consequently unkempt and not beautiful, has

> hayre . . . rekand na forthir na hir neke (Sc. Leg. 18. 225 f.),

or, according to another account, her hair is so

> þunne and schort þat it miȝte onneþe helie hire scholle.
> Horst. D. 39. 145.

The hair of handsome men should fall down over the shoulders, but must not be too long.[34] The Green Knight has " longe louelych lokkeȝ " (Gaw. & Gr. Kn. 419), the exact length of which is described as follows:

> Fayre fannand fax vmbe-foldes his schulderes,
> A much berd as a busk ouer his brest henges,
> þat wyth his hiȝlich here, þat of his hed reches,
> Watȝ enesed al vmbe-torne, abof his elbowes
> þat half his armes þer vnder were halched in þe wyse
> Of a knygeȝ capados, þat closes his swyre.   Gaw. & Gr. Kn. 181.

The hair of St. Bartholemew is of indefinite length, it being merely stated that

> His eres with hare er couerd all.   Horst. c. 24. 85.

When the hair of men, however, grows so as to become longer

---

[34] So on Old French, cf. Loubier, *op. cit.* p. 54. Among the South Germans of the 13th century the hair reaches hardly to the neck (Schultz, *op. cit.* p. 287); and in the Old Norse it comes to the lobes of the ears. Cf. Weinhold AL. 182.

than to the middle of the arms, it is considered very ugly.   An
exceedingly hideous giant has

> lokkes . . . longe the lenghe of a ȝerde (Mort. Arth. 3282),

and of an equally loathly forest-monster we are told,

> Unto his belt hang his hare. Iw. & Gaw. 253. (Comp. Lib. Des. 139, note).

Orpheus, after long wanderings, has rough hair and

> Benethe his gurdel [35] it is ys y-grow (Orph. 253; Orf. 498),

and of Beves become palmer it is said,

> And to his gerdel heng is fax. Bev. A. 2243 (Cf. Note).

Later Beves is placed in prison where

> þe her on is heued grew to is fet. Bev. A. 1537.

The Devil is described as having hair reaching to his feet,

> fowl hare duwne till his fete. Horst. C. 24. 310

(Cf. Sc. Leg. 9. 219; Horst. D. 55. 179: and comp. *Leg. Aurea,
crinibus ad pedes protensis,* Horst. *Leg'samml.* 9. 219.   Cf.
further Dest. Tr. 8787.).   Without reference either to beauty
or to ugliness is the description of an old hermit whose hair and
beard fall down to his feet, completely clothing his body.   Horst.
D. 36. 616.

Since hair of a certain length is considered so very beautiful
and a mark of dignity and position, to have it cut is the greatest
of dishonors.   As a part of the torture of St. Christine the Duke
commands his minions to

> kytt of hire tresse,
> Let noght of hire be brighte,
> And shaue hire hede.
> Horst. B. Misc. 6. 345. Cf. Boc. 3. 650: Sc. Leg. 7. 54; 45. 227.

Of one Bardulf, wishing to enter a rival camp unknown, we are
told,

> he lette sceren half his hæfd (Laȝ. 20309),

---

[35] On hair reaching to the girdle cf. Kölbing, *Engl. Stud.* XI, 499; Kaluza
to Lib. Des. 139.

to which the MS. Cott. Oth. immediately adds,

> ase mon doþ an fole.[36]   (Comp. Beryn, 2916 f.)

Robert of Cicyle, as a matter of penance,

> het a barbur him before,
> þat as a fol he schulde be schore,
> Al around lich a frere,
> An honde brede boue eiþer ere.   Horst. B. Misc. 10. 169.

(Cf. further Trev. IV. 61. 351; V. 368, 25.).   Cutting the hair is also a sign of servitude and submission to a conqueror. The women of a land subjugated by Arthur, in order to obtain his mercy,

> heore uæx fære
> wælden to volde,
> curuen heore lockes,
> & þer niðer læiden,
> to þas kinges foten.   Laȝ. 21873.

(Comp. Trev. IV. 88; ? Torr. 2212; and Chaucer, C. T., A. 215.).   A closely cropped head is decidedly ugly,

> Neptanabus in theo way stod,
> With pollid hed, and of his hod.   (Alis. L. 215),

or, as in the case of Chaucer's Yeoman, it is at least a sign of low birth; [37]

> A not-heed hadde he.   C. T., A. 109 (Cf. Skeat's note, vol. v. p. 12).

Bald.   That baldness of the head is no mark of beauty goes without saying, but only a few times is it given as one of the

---

[36] For cutting of the hair like a fool, cf. Gaston Paris, *L'Histoire Literaire de la France*, tome XXX. p. 231.

[37] So in the German, " Dem Unfreien war nur geschorenes, ungehindert wachsendes Haar nur dem Freien und dem Edeln gestaltet," Wackernagel, *op. cit.* p. 190.   In Old Norse thralls and dishonored women have cropped heads, Weinhold AL. p. 180.   And in Old Fr. shorn hair is ugly, cf. Loubier, *op. cit.* p. 54.   At the time of the Conquest the Normans wore short hair, because of which they were said to resemble priests rather than warriors (Cf. Trev. VII. 239).   It is reported of the men of Frisia that they " beeþ i-schore aboute, and euir þe more gentil man and noble, þe hiȝer he is i-schore."   Trev. I. 263.   For the original law requiring priests to shave, cf. Trev. v. 25.

characteristics of ugliness. Alexander meets an ugly man in the forest, of whom it is said,

> Caluȝ was his heude swerd   (Alis. L. 5950),

Machaon is " ballid as a cote " (Lyd. II. 4673; Dest. Tr. 3848), and of Chaucer's Miller we are told that his skull is " As piled as an ape." C. T., A. 3935, 4306. Judging from the remaining quotations, kings and monks seem to have been peculiarly subject to the misfortune of having bald pates.[38] Wm. the Conqueror is said to have been " ballede " (R. Glouc. 7731; Wm. Malms. 458; Trev. VII. 314) and Henry I is likewise afflicted (R. Glouc. 8841; Wm. Malms. 642.). Of the patriarch Jacob we learn,

> his heed was al bare for elde (Cur. Mun. 5165),

the Abbot Samson is *calvus fere omnino* (Joc. Brak. 29; comp. Wm. Malms. 671), and Chaucer remarks of his monk, rather humorously I think, that,

> His heed was balled, that shoon as any glass. C. T., A. 198.

Sometimes the condition of being without hair gives rise to the nickname " the bald." Cf. " Charles þe balled." Trev. VI. 299, 305, 317, 369, 429.

That hair should curl is absolutely essential to the beauty of both men [39] and women. Such highly appreciated ringlets are, for the most part, described as being crisp, L. *crispus,* tho they are sometimes said to be " crulle." [40] The hair of St. Bartholomew is

> swiþe crips, non mai cripsore beo, Horst. D. 55. 64.

---

[38] A legend writer gives the information that a preponderance of the element air " wole " make a man " balled sone." Horst. D. 45. 684.

[39] In Old Norse for men to have curly hair is considered effeminate. The hair of heroes hangs smooth and straight. Cf. Weinhold AL. 182.

[40] For many other citations cf. Murray, art. crisp and curled; Bos-Toll. art. *loc* and *wundenloc.* Cf. also Mabinog. p. 209. The man who has a preponderance of the element fire is crisp of hair. Horst. D. 45. 686. Compare Chaucer, C. T., A. 81, 3314, and cf. Skeat's note, Vol. v. 10, where he suggests that possibly curling tongs were in use.

It is the same in Gir. Cam. II. 68; Horst. C. 24. 86; Sc. Leg.
9. 49. Cf. further Trev. I. p. 53; III. 398; Dest. Tr. 3968;
Lyd. II. 4550; Dest. Tr. 3757 and Lyd. II. 4356; Horst. B.
Misc. 7. 277; Mort. Arth. 3352; Horst. D. 59. 182.

" Crulle " hair is not so common;

His hed was crolle. Alis. L. 1999.

Cf. lokkes . . . crolle, *ibid.* 4164; crollid her, Ferum. 1354
(O. F. orig. *poil cercele,* Feriebras, 2184) ; heer kurlyd semely,
Boc. 7. 185. Of the beautiful black hair of Ajax T it is said
that it

Serklyt of hom seluyn (Dest. Tr. 3780),

or according to Lydgate,

vpward ay gan folde,
In compas wyse, rounde as any spere. Lyd. II. 4584.

If curly hair is beautiful, then, by contrast, straight hair
should be ugly—and so it is. The short, white, unkempt hair
of St. Egipciane is also said to be " streke " (straight), Sc. Leg.
18. 225. We may also compare the description of Chaucer's
Pardoner;

This pardoner hadde heer as yelowe as wex,
But smothe it heng, as dooth a strike of flex,
By ounces henge his lokkes that he hadde,
And ther-with he his schuldres over-spradde,
But thine it lay, by colpons oon and oon. C. T., A. 675 ff.

Beautiful hair is also described as being fair, comely, and as
soft and shining as silk. Cf. Bödd. W. L. II. 13; Arth. & Merl.
5816; Alis. L. 163; Guy B. 58; Gower, V, 5464; Le Mort.
Arth. 805. Of Pyrchel it is reported,

Pyrchel had fair heued wiþ her,
þoru gift of kynde þat was er;
Som-what was hit fair out of kynde,
þat ȝut of his her write men fynde   (R. Brunn. 4057),

and Eurydice's hair no man could describe. Orph. 53. Of
Paris we are told that his hair was soft, " huet . . . as haspis

of silke " (Dest. Tr. 3899), and Polyxena's beauty is greatly enhanced by the fact that

> Here lovely ffax shyned as selke. Troy H. 1337.

As a sign of his great bravery, prowess, and strength, of Alexander it is said,

> þe fax on his faire hede was ferly to schawe,
> Large lyons lockis þat longe ere & scharpe. (Cf. Alis. C. 601 and note).

Beautiful hair is always nicely kempt,[41] parted in the middle,[42] and, in the case of women,[43] plaited in small tresses or braids and bound with golden or silken threads. In the description of Helen, we find,

> The shede þurghe the shyre here shone as þe lilly,
> Streght as a strike, straight þurgh the myddes,
> Deperted the proudfall pertly in two,
> Atiret in tressis trusset full faire. Dest. Tr. 3023 (Cf. Guido, sig. d₃).

The Christ had " a sheed biforn" (Cur. Mun. 18837); and Chaucer remarks of Absolon,

> Full streight and even lay his joly shode. C. T., A. 3314.

In Ferum. 5881 we find " ȝealwe traces & fayre y-trent"; and in Lyd. II. 4741, " her . . . Bounde in a tresse." Cf. further Alis. L. 207; Alis. C. 3450; Sev. Sag. 477; Lob. Frau. 48; and compare Chaucer, C. T., A. 1049, etc. To untress the hair seems to have been a sign of sorrow [44] (Sev. Sag. 477; Trev. III. 267), or of devotion (Chaucer, C. T., A. 2289). Beautifully tressed hair is often adorned with precious stones, (Awn. Arth.

[41] Comp. Chaucer, " Hir heer was kempt," C. T., A. 2289, 2142, 2134, 3374, etc. But cf. Skeat's note, Vol. v. p. 84.

[42] For parting of the hair in the middle cf. Hill, *op. cit.* p. 13. Among the Germans the hair is parted on the side, cf. Schultz, *op. cit.* I. 287.

[43] For full account of the modes of wearing the hair in England cf. Strutt, *op. cit.* II. 128 ff. Schultz (I. 287) and Loubier (*op. cit.* p. 58) both give instances to show that, in the M. H. G. and in O. F., men also wear their hair in tresses, but it is not so in English. In the Old Irish, warriors bind up their hair before going into battle. Cf. Leahy, I. 71. Comp. Weinhold AL. 183.

[44] To draw the hair is also a sign of sorrow, cf. Tars. 100; Iw. & Gaw. 823; Oct. N. 1715; Alis. L. 5876; Sc. Leg. 45. 121; Guy B. 7413, 7281; Gener. 6584, etc.

3

369), tiaras of gold,[45] or coronets of leaves and flowers (Chaucer, C. T., A. 2289.), or braided with roses and lilies (Bödd. W. L. V. 10). One particular head-dress may be mentioned; namely, the " horned " mode,[46] which is especially favored by the gay, and detested by the more serious minded.

One of the chief characteristics of an ideally ugly man is matted, disordered, and filthy hair.[47] The Devil is described as being "ragged and longe-tayled " (Horst. C. Misc. 12. 295), and in other places he is called a " feltured fende." Gowth. A. 74 (cf. note), 784; Emar. 563. Of an ugly giant it is said,

His fax and his foretoppe was feltered togederes (Mort. Arth. 1078),

and of another grisly monster,

Hys hed is row wyth feltred here, Ipom. A. 6147 (cf. note).

Sometimes the hair reaches right up to the eyes like that of a dog. Of the wicked Geoffrey, Arch. of York, the description runs, *facie canina, barba comaque infra supraque lumine tenus hispida tota* (Gir. Cam. IV. p. 420), and an ugly giant is

herede to þe hole eyghne with hyngande browes. Mort. Arth. 1083.

Coarse, rough hair is compared to the bristles of swine;

Hys heere was as þe brystels of a sowe, Bev. C. 2519;
Blake brysteld as a bore, Ipom. A. 6147 (Cf. Alis. L. 5768).

Sometimes the whole body is hairy, which gives rise to various comparisons with cows, sheep, hogs, and bears;

Rowgh they weore so a beore, Alis. L. 6124 (Cf. Alis. C. 4126, 4726);
There hy seighen men . . .
And wymmen as beres rowe,
Brestled hy weren as hogges, Alis. L. 5768 (Cf. Alis. C. 4746);
Al blak so cole-brond,
And rowgh as beore to the hond, Alis. L. 6260, 6368;
He was rughher than any ku, Alis. L. 5956;
Row he was also a schep, Bev. A. 996 (note).

Compare Cur. Mun. 3487; Dest. Tr. 7719.

---

[45] For woman's head-dress cf. Strutt, *op. cit.* Plate XCVIII.

[46] For an arraignment of the custom, cf. Robert of Brunne's *Handl. Synne*, 3223 f.; and for full history, cf. Strutt, *op. cit.* II. 129 f.; Hill, *op. cit.* I. p. 129.

[47] So in the Old French, cf. Loubier, *op. cit.* p. 56; Voigt, *op. cit.* p. 56; and in the M. H. Ger., cf. Schultz, *op. cit.* p. 220.

§ 2. BEARD

As in the case of hair, white, hoar, or gray beard [1] is mentioned as a sign of age, and is generally respected and venerated accordingly. St. Bartholomew is described as *barba prolixa habens paucos canos,* Gir. Cam. II. p. 68. (Compare his description in Sc. Leg. 9. 52; Horst. D. 55. 66.). Cf. further Gir. Cam. VIII. 279; Rol. & Vern. 80; Horst. C. Misc. 8. 696; *ibid.* Misc. 22. 138; Trist. 685; Guy B. 10821; Grail 15. 639; Guy A. St. 45. 10.

Where venerable old men are said to be hoar or white-hoar, the general description probably refers to the beard and hair together (cf. § 1.). Sometimes, however, the beard is directly described as being hoar (Arth. & Merl. 3677; Rich. 6822; Horst. D. 55. 66; Grail 15. 637; Ferum. 4236; Alis. L. 1596; Ferum. 84, 2202), gray (Ferum. 2233; Horst. C. 24. 91), gray-hoar (Ferum. 936, 708; Rol. & Vern. 663), or as white and hoar as the driven snow;

> And as blaȝt was his berd as any briȝt snaw, Alis. C. 4925.

(Cf. Lat. Orig. *barba tanquam purissima lana,* in Skeat's note to *loc. cit.*)

> And as a bussh which is besnewed,
> Here berdes weren hore and whyte, Gower, I. 2045.

The word "hore," meaning filthy, dirty, is used once in the description of the beard of a terrible giant,

> Huke-nebbyte as a hawke, and a hore berde, Mort. Arth. 1082.

That the word here does not mean hoar is suggested by the fact that eight lines below the same beard is described as being "brothy and blake." (Cf. § 1, note 28; and Holthausen, *Beibl. zu Anglia,* Aug. 1913, p. 251; § 2, note 6).

---

[1] Compare Chaucer's Franklin,

> Whyt was his berd as is the dayesye, C. T., A. 332.

For many other citations cf. Willms, *op. cit.* pp. 20, 22, 30, 28.

Beggars, palmers, pilgrims, and other very old men are generally described as having long, bushy beards:

> A begger þer com in,
> Wiþ a long berd on his chin. Arth. & Merl. 1932.

Cf. further Gir. Cam. v. 389; vii. 26; ii. 68; Horst. D. 55. 66; Sc. Leg. 9. 52; Cur. Mun. 5313; Guy C. 7913; Guy A. 6837; *ibid.*, St. 75. 7; Guy B. 7418, 7729 (pilgrim); Rich. 6822 (wise messengers); Sow. Bab. 2005; Rol. & Ot. 80, 277 (Charlemagne); Horst. C. 6. 234; Sc. Leg. 9. 218 (Devil); Trev. I. 354; v. 369; viii. 145; Beryn. 2440; Horst. D. 55. 177.

Long beards are definitely described as reaching to the knees, to the breast, to the navel, and even to the feet. Of a strange wonderful women we are told, *Duvernaldus . . . mulierem habebat umbilico tenus barbatam* (Gir. Cam. v. 107), and Alexander meets other women who have "berdis to þe pappis," Alis. c. 4116. Of an ugly forest giant it is said,

> And to his nauel henge his berd,
>   (Alis. L. 5951, 5599, 6749); Guy B. 3353).

and the terrible cannibal monster of Mort. Arth. 1090, has beard "þat tille his brest rechede." Of Orpheus on his wanderings we are told that his beard

> To his girdel stede was growe   (Orfeo, 256),

and some time later we hear that

> his berd hongeth to his kne   (*ibid.* 498)

Since both handsome and ugly men have long beards, it is almost impossible to determine just what length is most appreciated; but that a full beard is a sign of manly strength and vigor goes almost without saying.[2] Charlemagne is described

---

[2] Cf. Chaucer's Somnour with "piled berd" (C. T., A. 627), i. e. thin, stragly; and the Pardoner,

> No berd hadde he, ne never sholde have,
> As smothe it was as it were late y-shave   (*ibid.* 689.),

and the Reve,

> His berd was shave as ny as ever he can,   (*ibid.* 588),

All these quotations poke fun at men of low caste; at least the lack of beard is no sign of beauty.

as " havynge berde unto his feete of greate broodenesse " (Trev.
vi, 253), and of a fair wounded knight it is said,

> Hys berde was longe as a spanne,   Guy B. 4285.

The beard of Beves as a palmer " to is brest wax " (Bev. A.
2243), and of him later it is stated that

> Al þai seide, þat hii ne siȝe
> So faire palmer neuer wiþ eiȝe,   (*ibid.* 2245).

The great Green Knight has " A much berd as a busk " (Gaw.
& Gr. Kn. 182), the beard of Duke Neymes "was huge &
straȝte along " (Ferum. 2204), and in the army of Darius
there is said to have been many a powerful " long-berdet Bar-
baryn " (Alis. l. 1924). The god Ammon has a bushy beard
with thinly grown hairs,

> A berd as a besom with thyn bred haris,   Alis. C. 320.

To be beardless is to be the object of derision and mockery,
and to be called beardless is an insult. The Green Knight
taunts Arthur's men with being " bot berdleȝ chylder " (Gaw.
& Gr. Kn. 279), and Torrent is branded a " berdles gadlyng "
by the giant who is to fight against him, Torr. 1014. If, however, young men are valiant and full of prowess, they are all
the more wonderful because of being beardless. Walter,
Steward of Scotland, is still a great leader in spite of the fact
that he is " bot an berdlass hyne " (Barb. xi. 216), and to
arouse our especial admiration we are told of another knight
that,

> Yonge he ys and mekyll of myght,
> Berde hath he noon, þat nobull knyght,   Guy B. 11667.

The same disgrace is attached to shaving the beard [3] as to

---

[3] Giraldus remarks that the Welsh were accustomed to shave the beard
after the manner of Caesar's time, vi. 185. It is also said of the Abbot
Samson that he often shaved, Joc. Brak. 29. In Chaucer is found the
expression "to make a beard," meaning to cheat, cf. C. T., A. 4096; *ibid.*
D. 361; H. of Fame, 689. The expression is a literal translation of the
O. F. *faire la barbe*, to shave or trim the beard. Cf. Skeat's Chaucer, Vol.
iii. p. 258. Interesting is the expression "to put against the beard," to
throw up to, or accuse, cf. Trev. ii. 325.

parting with the hair.   When a knight wishes to enter the
enemy's camp unknown, it is said,

> His hed his berd he dide al shaue;
> Men wend a were a folted knaue,   R. Brunn. 9843.

(Comp. Trev. III. 397; R. Glouc. 3160; Laȝ. 20303 f.; Beryn.
2916).   Since a great beard is a sign of virility and strength,
the greatest ignominy, short of being vanquished, that can come
to a knight in combat is to have part of the beard cut off by
his opponent:

> And wiþ þe point of his swerd,
> He schaved Williams berd,
> And com þe flesch riȝt niȝ,   Lib. Des. 379 f.

In the combat between Cornyfer and Roland it is said that
the battle was fierce,

> Ac Roland kepede hym fram ys berd   (Ferum. 2999.),

the young Percival, who has just cut off a giant's head, is called

> ane unhende knave,
> A geant berde so to schafe   (Perc. Gal. 2094),

and Otuel taunts his enemy with,

> Suþen þi berd was ischue,
> þou art woxen a strong knaue,   Otuel, 1329 f.[4]

Lucifer burns off the beard of Naymes for which insult he is
killed with a blow of the fist, Ferum. 2240-45.   Cf. further
Sow. Bab. 2000-10; Ferum. 615; Ipom. A. 8087.   The beards
of kings are sometimes demanded in token of submission.
King Reance has discomfited eleven kings and with their
beards has purfled a mantle.   There being space for one more
beard, he demands that the great King Arthur send him his

---

[4] It is also an indignity to have the beard pulled or shaken.   Cf. Gir.
Cam. v. 389.   A young knight taunts an old man with,

> Then schall y hys berde so schake,
> That his neck schall all to crake,
> > Guy B. 11765, 8207.   Cf. Ferum. 2204.

as a sign of defeat and submission.[5] R. Brunn. 12456; Mort.
Arth. 1003; Malory, Bk. I, ch. xxvi.

Black. Black beard, if it is rough, filthy, and unkempt, is
considered very ugly. Cf. Gir. Cam. iv, 420; Parton. 7288.
Of a poor palmer it is said,

> Al rowe was . . . his chinne   (Trist. 685);

Orpheus, after wandering a long time, has

> here of his herd, black and rowe   (Orf. 256);

and the head of the Saracen whom King Richard has eaten
as "hog meat" has a "black berd" (Rich. 2188). The beards
of loathly giants are sometimes said to be as black as pitch, or
in roughness and coarseness like the bristles of a hog:

> His berde as pyche ys blake,   Ipom. A. 6156;
> His berde like bristullis of a swyne,   Bev. M. 2509;
> His berde was boþe gret & rowe,   Bev. A. 2509.

Of the giant Dynabrok, described just after a feast of children's
flesh, it is said,

> His bryn, his berd þer-wiþ al lothen   (MS. P. was broþen),
> & al to-soilled wyþ þe spyk   (R. Brunn. 12344),

and, under similar circumstances, the same giant is described
in Mort. Arth., 1090 ff. thus,

> His berd was brothy and blake, þat tille his brest rechede,
> Grassede as a mereswyne with corkes fulle huge.

That brothy [6] here and in the preceding quotation does not
mean stiff, shaggy as Perry supposes (Cf. Gloss), but rather
soiled, filthy, covered with grease and rags of flesh, is supported by reference to Brune's original,

> La barbe avoit et les guernons,
> Soillies de cendre et de charbons,
> (Soilliez de char cuite es carbons),   Wace, 1090.

---

[5] For history of this episode cf. Gaston Paris, *op. cit.* Vol. xxx. p. 244.
[6] For further discussion of the word cf. Holthausen in *Beibl. zu Anglia*
Aug. 1913, p. 251, where he derives brothy from O. N. *bráð*, fleshy, full of
rags of flesh.

In this connection may be mentioned the descriptive Latin word *fuscus*. According to Blümmner, the word means dark or black, and is applied to descriptions of a " Bart der die Haut nicht gerade vollständig bedeckt, sondern wie die sprossende, noch durchschimmern lässt, also nur verdunkelt," *op. cit.,* p. 99. The Bishop Baldwin *Erat igitur vir fuscus* (Gir. Cam. vi, 148) ; so was Duke Meiler (Gir. Cam. v, 324), which, however, the author of Conq. Ire. translates " a man of dark semblant," p. 99. Bishop Remigius is said to have been *colore fuscus, sed operibus venustus,* Hen. Hunt, p. 212.

Yellow. Beards yellow [7] in color are more common than those of any other color. Of a dwarf we are told,

> His berd was ʒelow as wax,　Lib. Des. 139.

Kaluza quotes, in his note to the above line, from a description of another dwarf found in Degree (ms. Auch. to which I have, unfortunately, not had access),

> Bothe his berd and his fax
> Was crisp an ʒhalew as wax, l. 743.

In the presentation of Beves as a fair palmer we find that

> His berd was ʒelu, to is brest wax　(Bev. A. 2243),

of a devil, which has been gilded over, " his lochkes ant his longe berd blikede al ogolde " (Marh. fol. 43. 21), and the people who drink of the water containing the dust of the golden calf have " Gulden berdes," Cur. Mun., 6620.

Brown. Like the hair, the beard of the Christ is said to have been of a nut-brown color;

> Forked feire þe chyn he bere,
> Berd & heed of on hew were,
> Note broun as I tolde ʒow ere,
> Metely heer was on his chyn,　Cur. Mun. 18843 f.

---

[7] Comp. Chaucer,
His heer, his berd was lyk saffron, C. T., B. 1920, and cf. Skeat's note Vol. v. 185. Cf. Kaluza to Lib. Des. 139; Kölbing, *Engl. Stud.* xi. p. 499 for further discussion of yellow beards.

We find also the adjective *beaver-hued* used twice in descriptions of great and handsome knights' beards:

> Brode bry3t wat3 his berde, & al beuer hwed,   Gaw. & Gr. Kn. 845.

Cf. " beueren berde," Awn. Arth. 257.

Red. Red beards are comparatively rare.[8] The Abbot Samson, at the age of forty-seven, is described as *paucos canes habens in rufa barba* (Joc. Brak., p. 29), and Frederick I was likewise a man *barba rubens, utrimque interfusa canities* (Gir. Cam., VIII, p. 279). An old knight has a " Rody berde " in Parton. 9401; the King of Persia has both hair and beard " huet as þe fire " (Dest. Tr. 3857), and Menelaus is likewise red bearded (Troy B. 805. Cf. Lyd., II, 4769 and comp. Guido, *capillos et barbam velut igneam rubicundum,* sig. e₂ recto 2).

Different emotions are sometimes expressed in connection with descriptions of the beard. Diocletian, in contemplation, " strok his berd " (Sev. Sag. 142); a poor pilgrim in sorrow " drewe hys berde " (Guy B. 7412); and at a lively banquet we are told that

> Swithe mury hit is in halle,
> When the burdes wawen alle,   Alis. L. 1163.

It was a sign of mortal terror when

> þe Sowdan quakede body and berd
> > (Oct. S. 1713. Cf. Horst. B. 5. 1020),

and he was likewise afraid when

> He bote hys lyppys and schoke hys berde,   Oct. N. 1070.

Anger is expressed by biting or mumbling in the beard. Ipomedon says to his enemy,

> thou getyste here nowght . . .
> Thow3e thou byght on thy berde,
> > Ipom. A. 6878 (Cf. note Horst. C. Misc. 22. 574.)
> Tho this lettre was rad and herd,
> Money on redid in the berd,
> And saide they wolde with him fyght,   Alis. L. 2943.

---

[8] Compare Chaucer's Miller,

> His berd as a sowe or fox was reed,
> And therto brood, as though it were a spade,   C. T., A. 552 f.

When the young Gamelyn is full grown, it is said that he
"bygan with his hond to handlen his berde" (Gamel. 82), and
finding thus that he is a man, resolves to right his wrongs.
(Cf. Skeat's note to l. 82).

The style of wearing the beard is rarely mentioned. In the
latter part of the fourteenth century, however, the forked
beard seems to have been in vogue. Chaucer's Merchant has
a "forked berd" (C. T., A. 269) ; and of the Christ it is said,

> Forked feire þe chyn he bere   (Cur. Mun. 18844),

which doubtless refers to the beard. Sometimes, as we learn
from certain illuminations, the beard was cut into three or
more points.[9]

§ 3. FOREHEAD.

In the case of both men and women a beautiful forehead
should be large, broad, high, smooth and without any wrinkles.[1]
The Christ is presented with

> His forhede feir, wemles in siȝt,
> Wiþouten wrynkul hit was sliȝt   (Cur-Mun. 18839),

one infatuated poet thinks his beloved's brow brighter than
moonlight (Bödd. W. L. V. 19. Comp. Chaucer, C. T., A.
3310, "Hir forheed shoon as bright as any day."), while
another poet finds concerning women that

> Wiþ eiȝe, forheued & nose tretis,
> Al beutes þai han in wold, Lob. Frau. 49.

---

[9] For full discussion of beards cf. Strutt, *op. cit.* I. 11 f.; Hill, *op. cit.*
p. 13. For beards with two points cf. Strutt, Pl. LXXV; with three points,
ibid. Pl. LXXVI. Comp. Skeat's Chaucer, Vol. v. p. 29 on forked beards.

[1] So everywhere else, cf. Loubier, *op. cit.* p. 73; Schultz, *op. cit.* I 213, etc.
Compare Leahy, "Brave his brow and broad," *op. cit.* p. 37. Cf. also Sec.
Sec. p. 228, "The forhede al rounde, harde witte; a longe forhede ouer
mesure, a slow witte; a quarre forhede of meen gretnys tokenyth feyrness
and corage." Cf. Chaucer's Gladnesse, "Hir forheed frounceles al playn,"
Rom. Rose, 860 (Fr. orig. *blanc, poli, sans fronce,* 870). Cf. Sec. Sec. pp.
222, 223, 230.

Cf. further *frons libera,* Gir. Cam. I. 349; Feyre forhede, Guy B. 58; frount & face feir to fond, Bödd. W. L. X. 15; forhede fare and brad, Sc. Leg. 33.390; forred brade, Sc. Leg. 34.20; large forhed, Alis. A. 179; his browis brad & mad rycht wel, Sc. Leg. 11.91; frount large, Mort. Arth. 3331; Gower, v. 6305; Horst. D. 27.1183; forhed he & brade, Sc. Leg. 19.70; Longe forhede and wele made, Guy B. 4290; browed ful bolde (knight), Awn. Arth. 385 (Comp. Chaucer, browes stoute, C. T., A. 2133). Of an especially beautiful type of woman it is said,

> He seth hire front is large and plein,
> Withoute fronce of eny grein,   Gower, VI. 769.

With these may be compared Chaucer's Prioress,

> But sikerly she hadde a fair forheed;
> It was almost a spanne brood, I trowe,   C. T., A. 154.

In addition to the large size and great breadth of the forehead, it must be lily-white or as fresh and white as the snow.[2] St. Margaret has a " Forheed lely-whyt " (Boc. I. 209), and of Helen it is said;

> Hir forhed full fresshe to be-holde,
> Quitter to qweme þen þe white snaw,
> ouþer lynes ne lerkes but full lell streght,   Dest. Tr. 3027.

A very narrow, low, or a very broad forehead is exceedingly ugly. Geoffrey, Archb. of York, has a typically " villainous low " forehead; he is *capite grosso, et tanquam simiam simulans usque ad cilia fere fronte pilosa,* Gir. Cam. IV. 240. " Hir front was nargh " is said of an ugly hag (Gower, I, 1683); and the brow of a forest giant " Was bradder than twa large span," Iw. & Gaw. 255 (Fr. orig. *plus de deux espanz de le,* Yvain, 298.). The cannibal giant in Mort. Arth. has a forehead covered with a thick, hard skin spotted or splotched like the hide of a frog;

> His frount and his forhevede alle was it over,
> As þe felle of a froske, and fraknede it semede,   Mort. Arth. 1080.

---

[2] So in Lat. cf. Blümmner, *op. cit.* 34. Cf. Willms, *op. cit.* p. 28 for O.E.

Another account of Arthur's combat with the same monster says that the Briton

> smot þen ssrewe in þe frount mid god ernest ynou,
> & þe vel & fless was so hard & þe scolle hard & þikke,
> þeruore þei it ne come noȝt þoru,   B. Glouc. 4227.

Wrinkles on the brow are a sign of age,

> þe frount frounseþ þat was shene   (Cur. Mun. 3571),

or they accompany physical exertion,

> þenne tas he hym stryþe to stryke,
> & frounses boþe lyppe & browe,   Gaw. & Gr. Kn. 2305.

§ 4. EYEBROWS.

The word which seems to express most forcibly and clearly for Middle English poets their ideal of beautiful eyebrows, is the adjective "bent." It describes the eyebrows arched or curved in the form of a strung bow, which the chronicler praises so highly in Eve, *prodit in arcum Forma supercilii,* Gir. Cam. I. 349. Bent brows, sometimes further described as being bright or like silk thread, are found as follows: "Ybend wex eyþer breȝe," Bödd. W. L. v. 18, 25; VII. 26; Lob. Frau. 34 (cf. Kölbing's note); Bev. M. 399; "Bryght browse ibent," Alis. A. 181;

> Her browes as selke þrede,
> Y-bent in lengþe and brede.   Lib. Des. 940;

Ferum. 5881, 1074; Guy A. 68; Parton. frag. 40; Gower VII. 4418; Squyr. 714. Boc. I. 210; Parton. 5155.

Not only are beautiful eyebrows curved, but the arch must be high.[1] The Abbot Samson is described with *superciliis in altum crescentibus,* Joc. Brak. p. 29. In Bödd. W. L. v. 25, the poet sings of his love,

> Heo haþ browes bend an heh.

---

[1] High eyebrows in O. Fr. are ugly, cf. Voigt, *op. cit.* p. 57.

That high eyebrows are appreciated generally is suggested by an interesting passage in Strutt (*op. cit.* II. 126), where he quotes from the Sloane MS. 2435, Brit. Mus. (13th cent.). A knight gives advice to his fair daughters in the following words, " Fair daughters, see that you pluck not away the hairs from your eyebrows [2] nor from your temples, nor from your fore-heads, to make them appear higher that nature has ordained." This much appreciated arch in the eyebrows is expressed in Scottish literature by the adjective " brent." The word is ex-ceedingly rare in early literature, being used with the plural " brows;" in later literature it becomes more common, where it is found in combination with the singular " brow." Now, Jamieson in his *Dictionary of the Scottish Language* says that in all quotations where brent, meaning high, straight, upright is used in combination with brow or brows, it " denotes a high forehead, as contradistinguished from one that is flat; . . . smooth, being contrasted with *runkled* or wrinkled." Murray (Dict.) gives a like general meaning to the combination, in spite of the fact that he elsewhere [3] remarks that " In M. E. brow is only eyebrow; there is no such sense as modern ' fore-head,' *frons,* which appears not long before Shakespeare's time and first in Scotch." Undoubtedly, I think the combination, brent brow,[4] in literature later than about 1550 does mean high, smooth, unwrinkled forehead; but in earlier quotations, where brent is used in connection with the plural, brows, the

---

[2] Comp. Chaucer,

> Ful smale y-pulled were hir browes two,   C. T., A. 3245,

and cf. Skeat's note, " partly plucked out to make them narrow, even and well-marked." Vol. v, p. 99. Murray quotes from Cornwallyes Ess. **xx.** (1601), " We will pull our browes, and indure any paine to imitate the fashion."

[3] In *Transactions of Philol. Soc.* 1888-90, Pt. I. p. 131.

[4] For many other quotations cf. Murray and Jamieson, articles, *brent.* Compare the following passage from the Aeneis of Gavin Douglas,

> From his blyth browis brent and ayther ene,
> The fyre twinkling, VIII. xii. 14.

(Cf. Vergil, *geminas oui tempora flammas Læta vomunt*, Bk. VIII.). This is the last appearance of ' brent brows ' in English literature.

combination means *high eyebrows*. It is true that in one passage, "Wythe browys brante," found in Isum. A. 248, so far as the context shows it may refer to either forehead or eyebrows; but in the Sc. Leg. 34. 19 f. it is certainly the latter that are brent. St. Pelagia is described,

> with teyndir fassone & forred brade,
> with browis brent and (ene) brycht.

Again, in the description of a fair lady, the poet says,

> A fairer saw I never none,
> With browes brent, and therto small,   Eger & Gr. 945.

Laing, the editor of the above passage, suggests " ? curved " as the meaning of brent, which is in part correct, since, if the last half of the description were applied to the forehead, the words " brent " and " small " would be contradictory. It is more likely that the poet is trying to say that the eyebrows are high-arched, and delicate, not prominent. (Cf. *supra*, 'like silk thread'). And, finally, in one passage at least the poet does not mean a high, smooth forehead, namely, in Dest. Tr. 3030 ff. Here the 'forhed' of Helen has just been described as being whiter than snow, having neither lines nor wrinkles (ll. 3027 f.). Then the author proceeds;

> With browes full brent, bryghtist of hewe,
> Semyt as þai set were sotely with honde,
> Comyng in Compas & in course Rounde,
> ffull metly made & mesured betwene,
> Bright as brent gold enbowet þai were.

This is a comparatively close translation of the corresponding passage in Guido. The *frons* has just been described as being snowy and smooth, after which the account continues; *Miratur etenim in tam nitide frontis extremis conuallibus gemina supercilia quasi manu facta sic decenter eleuata flauescere vt*, etc. sig. d$_4$ recto 1. It may be easily seen from this that ' browes brent ' is an attempt to translate *supercilia . . . decenter eleuata*. On the other hand, I have found only one place where high eyebrows are spoken of as being characteristic of ugliness. Gower (I. 1678) presents an ugly old hag with " hire browes hyhe."

Beautiful eyebrows are further described as being 'blissful and bright';

> Quene was I some wile brighter of browes
> Thene berelle or Brangwayne, Awn. Arth. 144;
> Wiþ browen blysful vnder hode, Bödd. W. L. x. 19.

Prominent, overhanging, rough eyebrows are considered exceedingly ugly. Of two hideously deformed men we are told,

> Longe & side her browes weren,
> And rauȝt al aboute her eren (Cur. Mun. 8079);

a giant is described "with hyngande browes" (Mort. Arth. 1183), and of another it is said,

> His browys full they hynge, Ipom. A. 6149.

(Cf. Kölbing's note to *loc. cit.,* and comp. Gir. Cam. vii. 279). A Saracen "Hound" has "browse brod and hore" (Tars 436), *i. e.,* large, coarse, and filthy (cf. § 1. note 28; § 2. note 6), and of the giant Dynabrok, just after a meal of children's flesh, it is said,

> His bryn, his berd, þer wiþ al lothen,
> & al to-soilled wyþ þe spyk, R. Brunn. 12344.

Ugly eyebrows are further described as being rough (Ferum. 1954, 4435, 4615; Bev. A. 685 and note; Bev. S. 2511), and once, in their length and coarseness, they are compared to little bushes (Iw. & Gaw. 261). The favorite object of comparison, however, is the rough hair or bristles of swine (sows), and the person, usually a giant, is made more terrible in his power by a description of the great space between the eyebrows. This space, which is not only a mark of ugliness but of strength, is sometimes one or two feet, sometimes a span in extent;

> Hys browys as brystelys of a swyn, Oct. S. 932;
> He bereþ on euerich browe,
> As bristelles of a sowe, Lib. Des. 1340 (cf. note);
> He was brysteled lyke a sowe,
> A fote he had bytwene eche browe, Bev. O. 2225; Bev. A. 2510;
> Two foot bytwene his browe,
> A span long þey were, Bev. S. 2511; Rol. & Vern. 480;
> Ferum. 4435.

Likewise a great space between the eyes is a sign of enormous strength and sometimes of ugliness.   Of King Arthur's skull found in his tomb it is said, *Os . . . capitis . . . capax erat et inter oculos spatium palmalem amplitudinem large continueret,* Gir. Cam. VIII. 129 (Cf. Trev. VIII. 65).   And of Goliath we are told,

> Bitwene his eȝen þre fote he hade,   Cur. Mun. 7447.

If eyebrows too far apart are not considered beautiful, neither are those that are joined together.   The space between the eyebrows should be small, white, and well-marked.   The ugly Neoptholomus is described,

> Bytell-browet [5] . . . þat aboue met,   Dest. Tr. 3824.

(Cf. Guido, *superciliis iunctis,* sig, e₂ recto 1).   Cressid has only one fault, namely, that her eyebrows are joined together;

> And saue hir browes Ijyneden y-fere,
> No man koude in hir a lake espien,   Lyd. II. 4787. [6]

-----

[5] Cf. Murray (Dict.) art. ' Beetle-browed,' "Having prominent brows . . . having black and long eyebrows."   Comp. Piers Plowman, A. v. 109,

> He was bitel-brouwed.

For full discussion of the etymology of the word cf. Murray in *Trans. Philol. Soc.* 888-90, Pt. I, p. 130 f.

[6] The whole passage is evidently taken from Chaucer,

> And save hir browes joyneden y-fere,
> Ther nas no lak, in ought I can espyen,   Troil. & Cres. v. 813 f.

(Cf. Skeat, Vol. II. p. 498.).   Joined eyebrows were considered a mark of beauty by both Greeks and Romans and all Oriental peoples; cf. J. Fürst, *Philologus,* LXI. p. 387 f.   In the description of Briseis the facial characteristic of joined eyebrows is first qualified as a defect in Tzetzes (1150), and in the Roman de Troie of Benoit (*ca.* 1160), those authorities interpreting their sources in accordance with the standard of beauty of their times. Cf. G. L. Hamilton, Supercilia Juncta, *Mod. Lang. Not.* XX. 80.   Cf. also G. P. Krapp in *Mod. Lang. Notes,* XIX, p. 235.   Since the 12th century joined eyebrows are considered very ugly, cf. Loubier, *op. cit.* p. 76; Weinhold DF. I. p. 226; Schultz, *op. cit.* I. 213.   This is probably due to the fact that physiognomists thought of this facial characteristic as a sign of a dark and gloomy disposition.   It was clearly so in Greek times.   Cf. Fürst, *op. cit.* p. 389.   The M. E. versions of this oriental physiognomy have also an unfavorable attitude toward this facial characteristic.   Cf. Sec. Sec. pp. 115, 230, 233; Philos. 2612.

The lyrist sings the beauty of his love, an especial characteristic of whom is that

> Heo haþ browes bend an heh,
> Whyt bytwene, ant nout to neh,   Bödd. W. L. v. 25 f.

One of the distinguishing marks by which another beautiful lady is to be recognized is that

> Shee hath on her nose, betweene her eyen,
> like to the Mountenance of a pin,   Eger. & Gr. 619.

Tho F(urnivall) remarks in his note to this passage that " Her eyebrows meet," still it seems evident that the poet is trying to say that they do *not* meet, and that the space between them is the size of a pin—probably white.

The color of the eyebrows is seldom mentioned. Black eyebrows,[7] as a characteristic of feminine loveliness, are found only twice. Of St. Margaret it is said,

> Her browys blake & hyr grey eyne   (Boc. I. 210),

and Giffroun's love is described;

> Her browes also blake as selke threde,
> Y-bent in lengþe and brede,   Lib. Des. 940.

It may be remarked that in the latter passage the poet is giving a comparatively close translation of the French original,

> Les sorcils ot noirs et vautis,
> Delgies et grailles et traitis,   Bel. Inc. 1525 f.

This combination [8] of black brows, blonde hair, red cheeks, and white forehead is found also in the German, where it is supposed by Wackernagel (*op. cit.* p. 165) to be " eine Verbindung von Gegensätzen, die den Eindruck der Schönheit reizvoll steigert." Twice brown eyebrows are described, tho in these

---

[7] In the Celtic black eyebrows seem to be highly appreciated both for men and for women; " her eyebrows were of a bluish-black such as ye see upon the shell of a beetle," Leahy, I. 13, 100; II. 155; " her two eyebrows were blacker than jet," Mabinog. p. 194, 187.

[8] Comp. Schultz, *op. cit.* p. 213, Vol. I; Loubier, *op. cit.* 74-5; Weinhold DF. I. p. 226 for the combination of blonde hair and black eyebrows.

passages " browe broune " (Bödd. W. L. II. 14; IV. 39; Parton.
5159) probably means black eyebrows as it does in the German
and Old French. Cf. Wackernagel, *op. cit.* p. 166; Loubier,
op. cit. 74; Schultz, I. p. 213. Ugly black eyebrows [9] are found
only once in the description of a shriveled old woman, where
it is said,

þat noȝt waȝ bare of þat burde bot þe blake broȝes,   Gaw. & Gr. Kn. 961.

Green. One instance of green eyebrows is to be found in
the passage where the Green Knight [10] delivers his challenge
to Arthur's court. Amid the general silence following, he
waits and

Bende his bresed broȝeȝ, blycande grene,   Gaw. & Gr. Kn. 305.

Red. In the particular field covered by this study red eyebrows do not occur, but in the Merlin cited above (§ 1. note 22)
an ugly dwarf has " browes reade and rowe " (p. 635), and in
the Old Irish there is one example.[11] When Cuchulain meets
the great Queen, it is said that " A red-haired woman sat in the
chariot, bright red were her eyebrows twain." Cf. Leahy, II. 37.

The eyebrows are sometimes found to be the seat of the facial
expression of anger, joy, and sorrow. To raise the eyebrows
is a sign of anger. Laȝamon says of the Britons in battle,

þer wes moni bald Brut,
þe hafde beres leshes,
heouen up heore bruwen,

---

[9] Comp. Chaucer, " scalled browes blake," C. T., A. 3245 (cf. Skeats's note
in Vol. v. p. 52) ;

Ful smale y-pulled were hir browes two,
And tho were bent, and blak as any sloo,   C. T., A. 3245.

Cf. also Blümmner, *op. cit.* p. 57.

[10] Tho the knight is dressed entirely in green, of his person only the
brows are expressly described as being green. It was an ancient folk-
belief that the devil was accustomed to let himself be seen in green clothing. Cf. Wackernagel, *op. cit.* p. 167. Hence the green clothes of the
tempter of Sir Gawain. But cf. Holthausen to Per. Gal. 277; Schick to
Temple of Glass, 299; and Willms, *op. cit.* p. 55.

[11] In Latin literature Blümmner finds only one instance of red eyebrows.
Cf. *op. cit.* p. 163.

i-burst an heore þonke, La3. 22281 ff.[12]

(Cf. Rol. & Vern. 174; Song. Rol. 402.)

On the other hand, Uther Pendragon in sorrow and perplexity "heng his breowen adun," La3. 18374.[13]

Eyelashes. There is only one passage in which the 'browes,' meaning eyelashes are described. Meriones is presented with,

All the borders blake [14] of his bright ene,   Dest. Tr. 3969.

(Comp. Guido, *oculorum vero eius orbes nigro fuerant colore perlucidi,* sig. e₂ verso 2). And the eyes of Helen are said to have been

> ffull sutelly set, Serklyt with heris
> On the browes so bryght, borduret full clene,
> Stondyng full stepe and stable of chere,   Dest. Tr. 3038.

(Cf. Guido, *Quorum pilorum etiam in proceritate modeste frenabant palbebrarum habene,* sig. d₄ recto 1).

§ 4. EYES.

The eyes of both men and women, to be considered beautiful, must be bright and radiant, and above all in color *grey*. In fact *grey* seems at times to have lost any definite color significance it may originally have had, and to be merely a synonym for beautiful or bright and radiant. Our first quotation [1] for grey eyes is found in the description of the Christ;

---

[12] Murray (Dict. art. brow 2) gives this quotation as an illustration of brows meaning eyelids, L. *palpebrae*. But cf. Wace,

> *Faces noicir, iels roellier,*
> *Sorcils lever, sorcils baissier,*   Brut, 1145.

[13] Cf. Jamieson 'Dict. art. brent' for an instructive and amusing account of the lowering of the eyebrows in sorrow. Egill, just returned from the burial of his brother, sings, "Grief made me let fall my eyebrows." But when King Athelstan gives him a ring of gold, he says, "My eyebrows have been quickly raised by the king."

[14] For black and brown eyelashes in Old Irish, cf. Leahy, I. p. 77, "Proud his glances and dark eyelashes Black as beetle his eyes adorn"; "brown the lashes were that slept her eyes above," *ibid.* I. p. 108.

[1] For other citations cf. Willms, *op. cit.* p. 32; Skeat to Chaucer, Vol. v. p. 17. One of the tokens of a great-hearted man is that he has "eghyn grey or broune, y-lyke a camail here," Sec. Sec. pp. 222, 232.

> Studfaste his loke & symple ay,
> His eȝen clere & somdel gray   (Cur. Mun. 18849),

and, following Him, come many knights and ladies of romance, history, and legend who likewise have grey eyes. (Cf. further Bödd. W. L. v. 16; Lob. Frau. note; Tars. 935, 14; Launf. R. 429; Launf. M. 809; Alis. A. 182; Gaw. & Gr. Kn. 82; Mort. Arth. 2963, 3791; Isum. 732; Sc. Leg. xi. 90; Awn. Arth. 356, 599, 594; Dest. Tr. 3772, 3921; Horst. C. Misc. 17. 669, 725; Ferum. 5881; Gower v. 2474; v. 6305; vii. 4418; Guy A. 282; Guy C. 71, 282, 283; Erl. Tol. 343; Thos. Ercel. C. 132, 634, 674; Gregor. A. 308; Gol. Gaw. 769; Boc. i. 210: Conq. Ire. 54, 88, 98).

In an attempt to express more accurately the exact color meant, the comparison ' grey as glass ' is sometimes used;.

> Her iȝen gray as glas,   Lib. Des. 943.

(Cf. Erl. Tol. 343; Isum. D. 248). Once the comparison ' gray as crystal stone is found,

> Hys eyen grey as crystalle stone   (Eglam. 861),

and Chaucer presents an additional comparison which, so far as I have been able to find, does not occur elsewhere;

> his eyen greye as goos,   C. T., A. 3317.

The exact color meant to be expressed by the term *grey* is not, however, what we today would call grey; rather it probably carries with it the idea of light blue, or a bluish-grey inclining to light green or yellow. Discussing the meaning of ' grey eye ' in Shakespeare's time, Malone remarks (in his edition of Shakespeare's Works, 1821, Vol. iv. 118), that " By a grey eye was meant what we now call a blue eye." [2]   The same

---

[2] This theory is supported by quotation from Cole's Dictionary (1678) where grey, when applied to eyes, is rendered *ceruleus, glaucus.* Cf. also Dowden's note to *Romeo and Juliet,* ii. iv, 47, where he says; " It is certain . . . that grey . . . means sometimes bluish. Cotgrave has ' *Bluard,* gray, skie coloured, blewish,' *Cæsius* is explained by Cooper, *Thesaurus* (1573) ' gray, skie colour, with speckes of gray blunket' (i. e. greyish-blue); *Glaucus,* says Cooper, ' is commonly taken for blewe or gray like the skie

affirmation may be made with equal truth of the meaning of grey eye in Middle English literature. Aelfric's Glossary [3] of the 10th century renders *glaucus* into *græg* (163. 24); another glossary of the 11th century renders *glaucus* into *glæseneage* [4] (*Ibid.* 416. 1); and the Epinal [5] Glossary translates *glaucum* into *hẹuui vel* grei (473). Similarly, three times the description *oculis glaucis* found in Gir. Cam. (v. 272, 303, 323) is translated "grey eghen" in Conq. Ire. (54, 88, 98). Undoubtedly, then, grey sometimes means *glaucus,* and *glaucus* is supposed to have the significance light-blue,[6] or what is sometimes called water-blue (cf. Blümmner, *op. cit.* p. 145). But that this light blue color shades into light yellow or green is suggested by other definitions of *glaucus;* in fact, light yellow, light green, and blue all seem to be for Middle English translators and glossary makers about the same shade of color. The Corpus Glossary (cf. Sweet, *op. cit.*) renders *gillus* (*gilvus*), grei, 967; a 10th century glossary (cf. Wright-Wülcker) renders *crocus, ƺeolu uel* græg, 215. 38; another of about the same time renders *ceruleus* i. *glaucus,* grenehæwen, fah, deorc (*Color est inter album et nigrum, subniger*), 203. 1; and still a fourth in the 15th century renders *glaucus,* gelu, 586. 38. Moreover, twice Trev. translates the description in Higden, *oculis glaucis,* into "ƺelowe eyƺen" (I. 145, III. 399), and the author of Alis.

---

with speckes as *Cœsius* is, but I thinke it is rather reddie.'" Cf. also Furness' note to *Much Ado About Nothing*, v. iii, 28.

[3] Wright-Wülcker, *Anglo-Saxon and Old English Vocabularies*, Lon. 1884.

[4] The meaning of this "glassy-eyed" and of the comparison "Grey as glass" becomes clearer when we consider that glass in those days was not so clear and pure as in ours. "The Gothic white glass varied from bluish-green to green, sea-green, greenish-yellow and yellow," *Archæl.* XLVI. 115, note a. "Similarly, there was a bluish-green (grey) like that of the olive, or (purer) of a field of wheat just shooting into ear." *Ibid. p.* 116.

[5] Ed. H. Sweet, *The Oldest English Texts*, EETS. O. S. 83.

[6] Cf. Century Dict. "bluish-green or gray; especially of the eyes, light-blue or gray (*L. caesius*), the lightest shade of eyes known to the Greeks. Of a pale, luminous, sea-green color; of a bluish-green, or greenish-blue." The adjective *caesius* in descriptions of the eyes carries with it the idea of ugliness in the Latin (cf. Blümmner, *op. cit.* p. 157); but that color is considered beautiful in the O. French, cf. Ott, *op. cit.* p. 95.

C. makes a like translation of his Latin original, *glaucus* (Cf. Alis. C. 603 and Skeat's note to 597 f.). In the description of Achilles (Guido, *oculis glaucis,* sig. e_1 verso 2), Lydgate renders the Latin original into " eyen glawke" (ɪɪ. 4551), where the word " glawke," which here makes its first and only appearance in English literature, evidently means blue or light green. (Cf. Murray).

In addition, the Middle English word *grey* probably means the same as the Old French word *vair* since it often replaces the latter word in direct translations. The " grey eyen " of Guy C. 72 translates " les euz uairs " of ᴍꜱ. Corpus Coll. 69 ; the description,

> Her iȝen gray as glas   (Lib. Des. 943),

reproduces

> Les oils ot vairs   (Bel. Inc. 1532),

and the " eȝene graye " of Ferum. 5881 describes the fair Floripas to whom is given " lex ex vairs " in Fierabras, 2014. Chaucer's description of Ydelnesse,

> Hir yen greye as a faucoun   (Rom. Rose, 546),

follows closely the Old French original,

> Les yex ot plus vairs c'uns faucons   (Rom. de la Rose, 543),

as does also his description of Mirthe,

> With metely mouth and yen greye   (Rom. Rose, 822),

where the original runs,

> Les yex ot vairs, la bouche gente,   Rom. de la Rose, 823.

Lydgate also in his description of Mercury (Reson and Sens. ed. E. Sieper), speaks of " Hys eyen gray " (1715), following the French, " De verdz yeulx " (fol. 8a). In Cotgrave *Oil verd* is rendered " a greye eye." These illustrations are doubtless sufficient to show that generally the word *vair* passes over into the Middle English word ' grey ' in descriptions of eyes. As to the meaning of *vair,* we may pass over the more or less irrelevant conjectures of a great number of commentators,[7] and accept that given by Ott (*op. cit.* p. 49), namely, *gris-bleu.* " Vair dans cette acceptation est un attribut des yeux, il designe des yeux non pas d'un bleu foncé, mais d'un bleu d'acier." [8] In conclusion, it seems to me that there can be little doubt regarding the meaning of ' grey eye ' in most of the places where it occurs in Middle English literature; L. *glaucus* (*caesius, ceruleus*), light blue, inclining to light yellow or green; [9] Old Fr. *vair,* grey-blue, or bluish-green. It is, however, worth repeating that sometimes ' grey eyes ' seems to be merely synonymous with ' beautiful eyes,' i. e. bright, brilliant, laughing.

Bright eyes are definitely spoken of with favor in Wm. Malms. (642), *oculis dulce serenis,* and in Dest. Tr. 2422, and Sc. Leg. 34. 21. The adjective ' clere,' meaning lustrous, glancing, also describes the beautiful eyes of both men and women. (Cf. Cur. Mun. 18851; Sev. Sag. 2783; Launf. R. 429; Sc. Leg. 16. 700; Alis. L. 6426; Lyd. II. 4920; Grail, 17.

[7] As illustrations cf. " les yeux vairs étaient ceux dont l'iris . . . était diversifié par des points, par des taches, par des irradiations d'une couleur différente," Houdoy, *op. cit.* p. 43; " eine unbestimmte, bunte, schillernde Farbe," Voigt, *op. cit.* p. 57; " die unbestimmte Buntheit des Augapfels," Weinhold, *op. cit.* DF. I. 226; " manigfarbig, bunt, buntgefleckt,' Loubier, *op. cit.* p. 77. In the succeeding pages Loubier gives no less than ten other conjectures with a like bearing. In the Renaissance the variant *verd* was misunderstood, and *green* eyes became the fashion in France, cf. Loubier, *op. cit.* p. 82; Houdoy, *op. cit.* p. 83. Likewise in England green eyes were highly appreciated, cf. Furness, Romeo and Juliet, III. i, 221; Dowden, Rom. and Jul., *ibid.;* Douce, *Illustrations of Shakespeare,* I. p. 47; II. 193: Furness to Mids. Night Dream, v. i, 333; and Cunningham, Mids. Night Dr. *ibid.*

[8] Roquefort, in his *Glossaire* (cf. Loubier, *op. cit.* p. 77), says, " On dit aussi yeux vairs, pour yeux bleus, parceque, comme dans la fourrure vaire, il sont parsemés de petits points blancs "; and Wright says (*op. cit.* p. 238), " *vair*—blue or azure."

[9] It is indeed not surprising that blue eyes should be appreciated since they are the distinguishing characteristic of Germanic peoples, cf. Wackernagel, *op. cit.* p. 204; Weinhold DF. I. 219; Blümmner, *op. cit.* p. 135, *caeruleus,* deep-blue eye. Compare also the Old Irish, " Her eyes were blue as a hyacinth," Leahy, I. 13; " eyes . . . blue centered," *ibid.* I. 92, 99; II. 37, 151; " gray-blue eyes," *ibid.* I. 147.

141; " yghen cler als es cristall," Iw. & Gaw. 900; " eyen schene," Bev. M. 399 ; Dest. Tr. 3036).

Stepe.   The adjective ' stepe,' when used to describe the eyes of beautiful persons, means bright, luminous, radiant, shining; when used to describe the eyes of monsters and ugly giants, it means burning, fiery.   Our first quotation is an illustration of the latter meaning.   The Devil has " twa ehnen steappre þene steorren ant þene ʒimstanes," Marh. fol. 44, a2.   (Comp. Dest. Tr. 7724).   For the most part, however, stepe [10] is descriptive of beautiful eyes.   (Cf. Tars. 14; Bev. A. 685; Dest. Tr. 3758, 3101, 3040; Isum. 248; Horst. C. 24. 88; Lyd. II. 4551, 4646; Grail, 13. 651).   Apropos of the passage,

> He lokyd vp steype starande   (Guy B. 7730),

Zupitza remarks (cf. note to *loc. cit.*) that ' steype ' cannot mean bright eyes here, but that it " seems to mean ' with fixed eyes.' "

In order to make impressive the splendor and brilliance of the eyes of his heroes and heroines, the poet compares them to stars,[11] to gems, and to shining glass.   Of Eve it is said, *Lucida sideras praetendunt lumina gemmas* (Gir. Cam. I. 349), St. Fremund has " sterryssh eyen lik Phebus of fresshnesse (Horst. C. Misc. 20c. 964), and the eyes of Helen are said to have been

> Shynyng full shene as þe shire sternys,
> Or any staring stone þat stithe is of vertue,   Dest. Tr. 3036.

---

[10] For further discussion cf. Cocayne to St. Juliana, EETS. 51, Intro. VI; St. Marh. p. 108; Skeat, *Specimens of English Literature*, note to XIV (B), 1014; Skeat's Chaucer, Vol. V. p. 244; *Engl. Stud.* XI. p. 285.   The most important citations are from St. Katherine, 309, 1647; Homilies, Vol. I. p. 456.   Comp. Chaucer, C. T., A. 201, 753.

[11] Comp. Chaucer, C. T., A. 266,

> His eyen twinkld in his heed aright,
> As doon the sterres in a frosty night.

For comparison of the eyes to stars, sun, and moon cf. Ogle, II. p. 130 f. Lydgate has also the comparison, " And hir eyen . . . Resemblede onto torchys tweyn," *Reson and Sens.* 1115.   Cf. Sieper's note to last line, and compare Ogle II. p. 133 for other citations of the comparison of eyes to lamps, torches, and flames in later English literature, and in Classical sources.   The metaphorical expression ' light of the eyes ' is also found, Sc. Leg. 24. 459; 38. 417; 45. 125; Horst. A. 3859.

(Comp. Guido, *oculos duorum siderum radios quasi gemmarum,* sig. d₃ verso 2; Dest. Tr. 3942 and Guido, sig e₃ recto 1). Of Aeneas we are told that his fair eyes

> Glemyt as þe glasse, Dest. Tr. 3942.
>> (Guido, *oculis hilaribus,* sig. e₂ ver. 2).

Piercing. Bright eyes are occasionally described as being piercing; *ocellis ... confossis,* Gir. Cam. iv. 420; " With persyng eyen," Lyd. ii. 4984. The heavenly eyes (cf. Gower, vi. 771) of the beautiful lady pierce the heart of her lover,[12] causing always great pain, and sometimes horrible death. This conceit is especially beloved by Lydgate. Of Cressid's eyes we are told,

> þei wer so persyng, heuenly & clere,
> þat an herte ne my₃t hym hym silfe stere
> Ageyn hir schynyng, þat þei nolde wounde
> þoru-out a brest, God wot, & bi₃onde, Lyd. ii. 3671.

(Comp. Guido, *oculis venusta,* sig. e₂ recto 2. Cf. further Lyd. ii. 3671; Horst. C. Misc. 21. 116; Lyd's *Temple of Glass,* 582; Chaucer, C. T., A. 1567).

Glad. Lovely, charming eyes are further pictured as being merry, lossum, glad, or laughing; " eyes full mery," Squyr. 714; " lussum, when heo on me loh," Bödd. W. L. v. 17; " Eyen right gladde," Parton. 9401. Lyd.'s *Reson and Sens.* 5374, 1548, etc. The faded lover laments the fact that in age her eyes must became dim and ' unglad,'

> And sih my colour fade,
> My yhen dimme and al unglade, Gower, viii. 2826.

As to the expression of the eyes, Lydgate says of Tantalus that he was " of his loke wonder amorous " (Lyd. ii. 4554), and Chaucer describes the Carpenter's wife as having a " likerous ye " (i. e. " wanton eye," cf. Skeat gloss.), C. T., A. 3244.

Eyes glowing like fresh coals or flaming as the fire are some-

---

[12] For further occurrences of this conceit in later English and in Classical literature, cf. Ogle, ii. p. 135 f.

times described.[13]   Of Frederick I. it is said that his *oculi ig-
nescunt* (Gir. Cam. viii. 279); Merlin makes a prophecy concerning Arthur that

> of his eȝene scullen fleon furene gleden   (Laȝ. 18862);

and of the Christ, seen in a vision, it is said,

> And bothe his Eyen . . . ferden there
> Also cleer brennenge As Ony Fere,   Grail, 15.311 f.

For the most part, however, burning eyes are attributed to horrible devils (cf. " aghen glared als any glede," Horst. C. 24.
309; Horst. D. 55. 178; Horst. C. Misc. 3. 203), and loathly
giants (Cf. Ferum. 4437; Mort. Arth. 1087; Grail, 37. 107).

The proud, bold glances of warriors in battle are often compared to those of wild animals [14] in fight.   Such flashing eyes
in the hero are highly appreciated, but in the enemy are considered loathly and grisly; in either case they are calculated
to inspire fear;

> þer wes moni bald Brut, þe hafde beres leches,   Laȝ. 22281.

Cf. further Laȝ. 1885; Guy A. St. 125. 10; *ibid.* St. 76. 7; Rich.
3463; 1795; R. Glouc. 590; Lyd. ii. 4770, 4920.   Two knights
come to do harm to Beves in prison but

> So loþeliche he gan on hem sen,
> þe twei kniȝtes were aferde   (Bev. A. 685),

the fierce Ferumbras glances scornfully on his enemy and
laughs (Ferum. 356), and Eurydice laments to Orpheus,

> Alas thy lovely yȝen tuo,
> Loken on me as man on fo   Orph. 109.

Such stern, flashing, proud eyes of noble warriors are sometimes
compared to those of a falcon.   Ferumbras, an ideal knight,
" lokede so þe facoun " (Ferum. 1074), and the fairest of the
Seven Wise Masters is portrayed, " With eghen faire als a fau-

---

[13] Also in the Latin, cf. Blümmner, *op. cit.* pp. 206-7.   Cf. also Wülfing,
Angl. 28, 33; Regel in *Anglia*, i. 233.
[14] Comp. Chaucer, C. T., A. 2131, 2171.

koun," Sev. Sag. 121. On the other hand the gentle, mild eyes of women are compared to those of a dove. Of the Virgin Mary it is said.

> As dowfes eʒe hir loke is swete, Cur. Mun. 9363.

Differently colored eyes, mottled or variegated are also described, but nowhere other than as a most wonderful occurrence. Of William II. the description runs, *oculo vario, quibusdam intermicantibus guttis distincto,* Wm. Malms. 504. This single occurrence of the word *varius* [15] need not detain us as to its meaning; Giles translates the passage, " different-colored eyes, varying with certain glittering specks " [16] (Cf. Trans. Wm. Malms. p. 341). The description in Guido sig. e₂ verso 2, *varijs oculis,* is translated by Lydgate as " Diuers eyes ay mevyng in his hed " (Lyd. II. 562, comp. Chaucer, C. T., A. 201), which shows that the word is understood to mean ' of different colors, variegated.' Several times Alexander appears with his different-colored eyes, one black and the other yellow; [18]

> þe two eyne of the byeryne was bryghttere þane silver,
> The toþer was ʒalowere [19] thene the ʒolke of a naye, Mort. Arth. 3282.

Cf. further Alis. C. 603; Trev. III. 399; and the O. F. in the gap in Alis. A. p. 210.

Red. Red eyes are a sign of wrath or tears, or they are pictured in descriptions of the strange and wonderful. Henry II is presented with *oculis glaucis, ad iram torvis et rubore* [20] *suf-*

[15] For full discussion of the word and its relation to the Old Fr. cf. Loubier, *op. cit.* p. 75.

[16] Comp. beautiful Etain in Old Irish; " is colour of eyes (that of) eggs of a blackbird," Leahy, II. 156, 155.

[18] Comp. " And one eye was of a piercing mottled gray, and the other was as black as jet " (ugly maiden), Mabinog. 209. Spotted or varigated eyes are said to be a sign of an evil or vicious man, cf. Sec. Sec. pp. 115, 233.

[19] For further mention of yellow eyes cf. Chaucer, C. T., A. 2131, 2167 ('bright citryn'); Trev. I. 145. Cf. "And tho that haue eyen not wel blake, but declynynge to yelow, bene of good corage," Sec. Sec. p. 230.

[20] So in the Latin, *ruber* describes eyes red from anger, sickness, or loss of sleep, cf. Blümmner, *op. cit.* p. 164. Comp. Chaucer, C. T., A. 2131; and Sec. Sec. " he that hath rede sparkelynge eyen, his fierse and corageous " pp. 230, 233, 236, 115; Philos. 2602 f.

fusis (Gir. Cam. v. 303; Conq. Ire. 88), and to make the Green
Knight appear more terrible and wonderful, we are told that
" runischly his rede ygen he reled aboute," Gaw. & Gr. Kn. 304.
We may compare Chaucer, C. T., A. 2901,

> With slakke pas, and eyen rede and wete.[21]

Black.   Eyes of ugly people, when the color is given at all,
are generally described as being black.   Both Hugh de Laci
and Geoffrey, Archb. of York, ideally ugly men, are presented
with *nigris ocellis et confossis* (Gir. Cam. v. 354; iv. 420), and
Meiler with *oculis nigris et torvis* (Gir. Cam. v. 324; Conq.
Ire. p. 99).   A hideous giant has " blake yghen " (Oct. S. 935.
Cf. Guy. A. St. 76. 7; *ibid.* St. 125. 10), and the blackness of
the eyes of a terrible, ugly people is compared to ink (Alis. L.
6418).   Once the comparison ' coal-black ' is found,

> þin egen beoð colblake and brode,
> Right swo heo weren i-peint mid wode,   *Owl and the Nightingale*, 75.

Tho black eyes are generally considered ugly, yet in a few cases
they are described with great approval.[22]   Of one fair lady it
is said,

> On heu hire her is fayr ynoh,
> hire browe broune, hire eye blake   (Bödd. W. L. ii. 13 f.),

and of a handsome wounded knight we are told that

> Hys eyen were black, hys vysage brade,   Guy B. 4289.

Brown eyes,[23] in the description of a beautiful woman, are
found only once;

> Har rode was red, her eyn wer browne,   Launf. M. 242.

---

[21] For other citations of red eyes from weeping cf. Willms, *op. cit.* pp. 45,
48.   Cf. also p. 26 for ' white eyes.'

[22] For other beautiful black-eyed ladies cf. M. P. Tilly, The White Hand
of Shakespeare's Heroines, *Sewanee Review*, xix. p. 211.   Women with
golden hair and black eyes are common in Spanish, Italian, and Classical
poetry; cf. Ogle i. p. 240; ii. 126, note 1.   Comp. two items in the description of a good appearance;

> In eyen and heerys havyng blaknesse,   Philos. 2552.

The ninth token of a good complexion is that a man should have " blake
eighyn othyr broune," Sec. Sec. pp. 223, 115, 114, 229.

[23] Brown eyes are a token of a good complexion (Sec. Sec. 223), or of
truth and justice (Philos. 2589).

Size. Large, round, and wide-open eyes are an especial mark of beauty. Cf. *oculis grossis . . . et rotundis,* Gir. Cam. v. 223 (cf. Conq. Ire. 98); *oculi grandes,* Gir. Cam. II. 16; x. 18; Horst. D. 55. 65; Bödd. W. L. v. 16; x. 18; Alis. L. 182; Sc. Leg. 9. 51; Guy B. 7408; Dest. Tr. 3821, 3772; Awn. Arth. 356; Guy. C. 5790; Lyd. II. 4551; Conq. Ire. 88; 'eighen apert,' (wide open), Alis. L. 5074. Certain men who have just been raised from the dead have eyes large with wonder, Cur. Mun. 17837.

Exceedingly large eyes, however, are considered very ugly. Devils and monsters are generally fitted out with glowing eyes, large and broad enough to be compared to saucers and basins. The devil who assails St. Margaret has eyes " brad as bascins " (Marh. fol. 44), ugly deformed men have also " eyen brad " (Cur. Mun. 8081), and terrible masks, worn to scare the enemy, are pictured

> With eghen that war ful bright and clere,
> And brade, ilkone, als a sawsere, Sev. Sag. 2783.

Of a loathly giant the poet says,

> As two dobelers euery eye he hathe, Ipom. 6157.
> (Cf. Horst. C. 24. 309.)

On the other hand small, deep-set eyes are equally as ugly as excessively large ones. Gir. Cam. draws Hugh de Laci with *nigris ocellis comfossis,* Gir. Cam. v. 354 (cf. IV. 420); a giant has " eȝene depe " (Ferum. 4437), and of another who is ' lyker a deuyl than a man' it is said that " His iyen were holowe," [24] Bev. O. 2227. Gower tells us of an ugly hag that she is shrunken and shriveled,

> Hire yhen small and depe set, Gower, I. 1679.

(Comp. Chaucer, ' with eyen narwe,' C. T., A. 625). Bulging, outstanding, pop-eyes are also no mark of beauty. Chaucer says of his Pardoner that

> Swiche glaringe eyen hadde he as an hare, C. T., A. 684.

---

[24] Cf. Kölbing to Ipom. 6157; comp. Seg. Melyn. 415, and Chaucer, C. T., A. 1362.

Judging from a few quotations, squint-eyed persons are not greatly admired. In fact squinting may be looked upon as a serious blemish. When Jacob goes to work in Laban's field for Rachel, it is said that,

> þe elder sister he forsoke,
> For she gliȝed seiþ þe boke [25]   (Cur. Mun. 3862).

We are at first somewhat surprised to find that the author of Dest. Tr. consistently defames Tantalus, Cassandra, and Aeneas by the statement that they also " gleyit a litell," Dest. Tr. 3772, 3995, 3942. But that he is not here writing with malice aforethought is suggested by the fact that he simply misunderstands Guido's description, *oculis varijs,* (sig. e_1 ver. 2; e_2 ver. 2; e_3 recto 1).

Rheumy, bleared eyes are of course ugly.[26] In the description of an ugly old woman we are told,

> þat noȝt waȝ bare of þat burde bot þe blake broȝes,
> þe tweyne yȝen . . . sellyly blered,   Gaw. & Gr. Kn. 961
>   (Cf. Horst. A. 3. 224).

Finally, we find certain prodigies and strange peoples who have sometimes one eye (cf. Alis. L. 5954, 4974; Torr. 1026; Dest. Tr. 13206; Barb. v. 506), sometimes three eyes (cf. Chaucer, Troil. v. 744), sometimes as many as four or more (cf. Alis. L. 6343; Horst. C. p. 494, 1. 183). Another people are described as being wall-eyed and able to see as well as cats by night (Alis. L. 5274, 6331), and Alexander is taunted with being " wald-eȝed " (Alis. C. 608), which probably refers to his having eyes of different colors (cf. Skeat's note to *loc. cit.*).

---

[25] What ' þe boke ' does say is, *Sed Lia lippis erat oculis,* Vulgate, cap. XXIX. 17; or according to Wycliffe's translation, " but Lya was with blerid eyen."

[26] Cf. Murray, art. ' bleared ' for other citations. The expression ' to blear the eye ' is also found in the sense of ' to deceive, to blind, to hoodwink, throw dust in the eyes,' cf. Rich. 3707; Oct. S. 1217, 1387; Ferum. 507 (cf. note); Lib. Des. 1523; Sev. Sag. 2952: Beryn. 445.

§ 5. NOSE; NOSTRILS.

A beautiful nose should be well set on the face, neither too large nor too small but in all manner well proportioned, slender, straight (' even '), high, and of a graceful length.[1] Again Eve leads all others in beauty,

> *Naris naturae vultum supereminent arte,*
> *Nec trahit hanc modicam, nec nimis in vitium,* Gir. Cam. I. 349.

In the chronicles other historical personages are described as follows; *naso eminente,* Gir. Cam. II. 68; *nares aequales et erectae,* Joc. Brak. 29; *naso adunco pertenui,* Hen. Hunt. 87; *naso mediocriter elato,* Gir. Cam. v. 323 (Cf. Conq. Ire. 98). If the nose is not naturally high and erect, it should be shaped thru artificial means. Giraldus tells us that this English custom was not known among the Irish peoples; *non enim abstetrices aquae calentis beneficio vel nares erigunt,* Gir. Cam. v. 150.

In the romances and legends are likewise conventional and rather indefinite descriptions. Cf. ' hire neose ys set as hit wel semeþ,' Bödd. W. L. v. 28; ' nose well sittyng,' Guy C. 68; ' Hyr nose was comely,' Bev. O. 401; Cur. Mun. 18841; ' nose namelich faire,' Alis. A. 185; ' Hir nose was streiȝt and riȝt,' Lib. Des. 942; Boc. I. 211; ' euene nose i-streiȝt a-doun a-long,' Horst. D. 55. 65; Horst. C. 24. 89; Gower, VI. 772; ' nose . . . at all maner ryght,' Erl. Tol. 344. A beautiful nose is sometimes described by means of the word ' tretys '[2] (cf. ' nose tretis,' Lob. Frau. 49; Chaucer, C. T., A. 152), which according to Cotgrave means slender and long; " *Traictif, nez traictif,* A pretty, long nose, a nose of graceful length." Of Helen it is further said,

---

[1] So in the Old Fr. cf. Loubier, *op. cit.* p. 89 f.; Voigt, *op. cit.* p. 59; also in the German, cf. Weinhold DF. I. p. 226; Schultz, *op. cit.* I. 214. In the Old Norse " eine hohe und grade Nase war nicht bloss schön, sondern auch adlig, die kurze und eingedrückte aber gemein," cf. Weinhold AL. 32. So also in the physiognomies, cf. Sec. Sec. pp. 115, 228; Philos. p. 83.

[2] Cf. Loubier, *op. cit.* 89; Herrtage to Ferum. 5883; J. L. Livingston, *Simple and Coy, Anglia,* XXXIII. 441; Gautier, *op. cit.* 276.

> Hir nose for the nonest was nobly shapyn,
> Stondyng full streght & not of stor lenght,
> Ne to short for to shew in a shene mesure,   Dest. Tr. 3041.

A high, hooked nose is very ugly,[3] being often compared to the beak of a hawk or an owl. The devil has a " hehe hokede neose " (Marh. fol. 44, a4), a hideous giant has a " nebe as an owle " (Ipom. A. 6162), and another monster is " Huke-neb-byde as a hawke" (Mort. Arth. 1082). Cf. Ipom. 6154; Horst. A. 3. 225; Cur. Mun. 3572. Neither very long nor crooked noses are appreciated. The Devil is " Croked . . . boþe nose and mouth " (Horst. D. 55. 183), Vernagu has a nose " a fot & more " in length (Rol. & Vern. 479), and certain masks are made more hideous by having " long noses" (Sev. Sag. 2781).

On the other hand, a flat nose is considered a great disfig-urement.[4] Cf. " fuatted nose, that is wrong," Alis. L. 6447 (Fuatted, flatted, Weber) ; " Nase bass," Gower, i. 1678. The French word *camus*[5] is occasionally borrowed to describe flat-nosed, snub-nosed persons. The giant Alagolafre has a " nose cammus," Ferum. 4437. Cf. Gower, v. 2479; Chaucer, C. T., A. 3934, 3974. The comparison to the nose of a cat is found twice. The nose of a wonderful forest man is " cutted als a cat " (Iw. & Gaw. 60), and the only defect that can be found in one noble knight is that he also has a " nose as a cat " (Arth. & Merl. 8716).

Nostrils. Wide-open, distended nostrils which generally ac-company a flat, snub nose are considered ugly;[6] those that are

[3] Comp. Sec. Sec. 228, 115; Philos. 83; cf. Wohlgemuth, *op. cit.* 30, 82: Loubier, *op. cit.* p. 90, etc.

[4] Comp. Malory, Bk. iv. ch. 8; Mabinog. 209; cf. Loubier, *op. cit.* 90; Voigt, *op. cit.* 59; Wohlgemuth, *op. cit.* p. 31; Weinhold AL. 32; Schultz, *op. cit.* i. 221. Comp. Sec. Sec. pp. 115, 228; Philos. p. 83.

[5] Cotgrave gives " *Camus*, flat-nosed, *Camuser*, to flatten, or quash down the nose, to break the bridge of the nose." Cf. Herrtage to Ferum. 4437; Skeat's Chaucer, Vol. v. 117; Philos. p. 83.

[6] Comp. Chaucer's Miller,

> His nose-thirles blake were and wyde,   C. T., A. 554;

Mabinog. p. 209; Cf. Loubier, *op. cit.* 90; Voigt, *op. cit.* 59; Wohlgemuth, *op. cit.* 31.

even, and neither too large nor too small are beautiful.   Both
Hugh de Laci and Geoffrey Archb. of York are described with
naribus simis (Gir. Cam. v. 354; iv. 420).   St. Bartholomew
has "ewyne ness-thrilles" (Sc. Leg. 9. 51), and the lovely
Helen is described,

> With thrilles noght thrat but thriftily made,
> Nawther to wyde ne to wan, but as hom well semyt,
>
> Dest. Tr. 3044.[1]

§ 5.   EARS.

I have failed entirely to find any mention of beautiful ears.[1]
Even in such detailed catalogues of feminine charms as are the
descriptions of Eve and Helen the ears are omitted, probably
because they are supposed to be covered with the hair of the
head.   But ugly ears are undoubtedly huge, large as those of
an elephant, hanging down on either side sometimes to the
girdle.[2]   Of the cannibal monster in Mort. Arth. 1086 it is
said,

> Erne had he fully huge, and ugly to schewe.   (Cf. Iw. & Gaw. 257).

The people Auryalyn are ugliest and most wonderful of all in
having ears large enough to shield them from the sun and rain;

> Eren they haveth an ellen long,
> That byneothe theo gurdel hit hongith,
> Whan hit snywith, other rayneth,
> Other theo sonne to hote schyneth,
> Anon ryghtis, his eren with
> Al his body he bywryeth,   Alis. L. 6448.

---

[1] For snoring as a sign of heavy sleeping, cf. Rol. & Vern. 629; Sc. Leg.
46. 225; Barb. vii. 190; Rich. 4229.   To pull the nose is a great indignity
and insult, cf. Torr. 1014.

[1] Also rare in other literature, cf. Loubier, *op. cit.* p. 91 (one instance);
Schultz (*op. cit.* i. p. 216) produces two examples of small, round ears,
as white as ivory; and Blümmner (*op. cit.* p. 34) finds that *niveus* is used
to describe beautiful ears in the Latin.

[2] Comp. Chaucer, C. T., D. 954; Sec. Sec. pp. 116, 229; Philos. 81; and
cf. Loubier, *op. cit.* p. 91; Voigt, *op. cit.* p. 60; Kölbing, *Engl. Stud.* xi. 504.

§ 6. MOUTH, LIPS, BREATH.

To be beautiful the mouths of fair women should be well-formed, well-proportioned, 'lovely' and 'fair.' With the single exception of the Christ no description of the mouth of a handsome man is found; and of Him it is merely said that his mouth was "feire ordeyned" (Cur. Mun. 18841). In descriptions of women cf. 'louely mouth,' Bev. O. 402; 'a mury mouht to mele,' Bödd. W. L. v. 37; 'mouth meete þertoo moste for to praise,' Alis. A. 184; 'Mouth . . . schapen . . . at all maner ryght' Erl. Tol. 344; 'Feyre mowthe,' Guy B. 58 ; Cur. Mun. 9359.

Lips. Beautiful lips are said to be sweet, gracious, small and laughing, soft and pleasant to kiss, and in color red [1] or ruddy. In descriptions of fair women cf. 'lyppes swete,' Bev. O. 401; Troy H. 1417; 'gracious lippes,' Alis. A. 182; 'lyppes small laȝande,' Gaw. & Gr. Kn. 1205; 'lippes softe,' Gower, IV. 3107; v. 5592; 'lefly rede lippes,' Bödd. W. L. v. 38; Gower, II. 385; IV. 774; Lyd. IV. 587; Parton. 5180; 'rosyn lippis rede,' Lyd. II. 4985; 'Hir lippes were louely littid with rede,' Dest. Tr. 3988; 'lyppys rody,' Boc. I. 212. Trevisa speaks of an image of Venus so craftily made "þat in þe mouþe and lippes, that were as white as eny snow, semede fresche blood and newe," Trev. I. p. 225. The exquisite complexion of Helen extends quite up

> To the lippus full luffly, as by lyn wroght,
> Made of a meane vmb þe mowthe swete,
> As it were coruyn by crafte, coloured with honde,
> Proporcionet pertly with painteres deuyse, Dest. Tr. 3049 f.[2]

---

[1] Comp. "her lips delicate and crimson," Leahy, I. 13; "Red as coral, her lips shall be smiling," *ibid.* I. 92, 100. Chaucer does not fail to have his customary joke at the expense of the conceit;

> His lippes rede as rose, C. T., B. 1916.

For the same appreciation of red lips in the Latin cf. Blümmner, *op. cit.* pp. 187, 163, 200, 202, 207. Cf. also Ogle II. 146 f; Willms, *op. cit.* p. 44; and Chaucer, C. T., A. 153, 3261.

[2] Here the author is again following Guido, but he omits the very important item that *ad oscula auidis affectibus inuitabant*, sig. d₄ rec. 1.

Kisses. To kiss the soft lips of the beloved one is great bliss; the touch of her mouth is sweeter than honey and the honeycomb, and all the spices of the South are not to be compared to it (cf. Lob. Frau. 177 f.). A lovesick swain laments to his lady,

> A suete cos of þy mouþ be my leche (Bödd W. L. XII. 12),

and another thinks that man fortunate who " hire comely mouth . . . mihte cusse " (*ibid.* VII. 27). Not the least of the charms of the fair Felice is said to have consisted in

> The mouthe so wele sittyng, ywys,
> To kisse it ofte it was grete blys, Guy C. 69 (Cf. Gower, v. 5592).

Breath. Moreover, the breath of the fair one is like the fragrance of nectar, and is sweeter than the perfume of the lily or the rose or of any other flower that springs on the heath (Lob. Frau. 166). Giraldus Cambrensis sums up the whole matter in his poetical description of Eve; *Mollia labra rubent . . . Oscula mel sapiunt, nectaris exit odor . . . os roseum, labra mollia, succus in illis Dulce sapit, sapiunt oscula pressa favum,* Gir. Cam. I. p. 349.

As for the lips of men, they are described only twice. The Abbot Samson is presented with *labiis grossis* (Joc. Brak. 29), and in the description of the King of Inde Chaucer speaks of " His lippes rounde," C. T., A. 2168.

Large,[3] wide crooked mouths are considered exceedingly ugly, being sometimes compared to those of mares, flat-fishes, boars, and hounds. For the most part, only the mouths of devils, giants, dwarfs, and other misbegotten monsters are thus described. Hideously deformed men have " muthes wid " (Cur. Mun. 8081. Cf. Alis. L. 6420, 6816; Sev. Sag. 2781; Bev. O. 2228; Horst. B. Misc. 6. 475), certain cannibal people " were mowthed so a mare " (Alis. L. 6125), the Garraniens have mouths " from that on ere to that othir " (Alis. L. 6466), one " floke-mowthede schrewe " (Morth. Arth. 7780) is as

---

[3] Comp. Chaucer's Miller with his mouth as great as a furnace, C. T., A. 559. Cf. Sec. Sec. 234.

." fflatt mowtheed as a fluke with fleryande lyppes " (*ibid.*
1088), while of another we are told that " His mothe wrythis
all way," Ipom. 6155. The mouth of the Devil, of course,
" ȝened wide " (Horst. C. Misc. 3. 203), and one most unfortu-
nate demon " Croked was boþe nose and mouth " (Horst. D. 55.
183). The god Ammon appears with " A mouthe as a mastif
hunde unmetely to shaw " (Alis. C. 321), and as usual Dame
Ragnell bears away the prize for ugliness in having

> A mowthe fulle wyde, and fowle igrowen
> With grey herys many on, Wed. Gaw. 533.

Ugly lips are those that are large, protruding, standing wide
apart, and so heavy that they hang down over the chin.[4]   Sometimes the lower lip is said to hang down to the navel,

> Heore nether lippe is a foul fother,
> For to the navel down scheo hongith,
> And foule al so carayne fongith   (Alis. L. 6467) ;

sometimes to resemble a blood pudding,

> Euery lype, I dare avowe,
> Hyngyth like a blode puddynge   (Ipom. A. 6151 and note) ;

or to be of such enormous size that the flesh of it lies in uneven
folds, each fold twisting itself out like an outlaw,

> And alle falterde þe flesche in his foule lyppys,
> Ilke wrethe as a wolfe-hevde, it wraythe owtt at ones,
> > Mort. Arth, 1092.

Cf. further Wed. Gaw. 555 ; Gaw. & Gr. Kn. 961 ; Gower, I.
1683 ; Bon. Flor. 94.

Grinning lips are horrible to look upon and as such are attributed to the Devil and his children.   Of the wicked and deformed Geoffrey, Archb. of York, we are told that his chin was
bent back which accorded well with *simulato . . . risui et ficto
continuoque fere oris rictui, quem in dolo praeferebat,* Gir.
Cam. IV. 420.   The cannibal monster in Mort. Arth. has " fleryande lyppes " (1088, 2779) ; the Saracen's head in Rich. is

---

[4] Comp. "And he þat hauys greet lyppes ys ffoltysch," Sec. Sec. pp.
115, 228, 234.

described, whose "lyppys grened wyde" (3189); and devils almost always appear to their victims "ʒellinge and grennynge" Horst. A. 4c, 198, 118, 443. (Cf. Sc. Leg. 12. 444; Horst. C. 6. 127; Horst. D. 43. 15; 15. 56; 23. 36; 45. 288, 799; 55. 104). The giantess Alagolafre's wife "grenned like a develle of helle," Sow. Bab. 2948.

§ 7. TONGUE.

I find tongues described only three times. The horrible devil who appears to St. Margaret has a tongue so long that he can swing it all about his neck; "his tunge swa long þat he swong hire al abuten his swire" (Marh. fol. 44, a8). Ugly masks worn to frighten away the enemy are described,

> With brade tonges and bright-glowand
> Als it war a fire-brand (Sev. Sag. 2785),

and Alexander meets an ugly people whose tongues in their wide mouths are like shingles or billets of wood;

> And a tonge as a schyde,[5] Alis. L. 6421.

§ 8. TEETH, GUMS.

Beautiful teeth of both men and women must be well-cleansed, well-proportioned and evenly set, and above all as white as ivory or as whale's bone.[1] Giraldus Cambrensis mentions in terms of the highest praise the well-kept teeth of the Welsh people, *quos assidua coryli viridis confricatione, . . . tanquam eburneos reddunt,* Gir. Cam. vi. 185. For the most part beau-

---

[5] A. S. *scid*, O. H. Germ. *scit*, M. H. G. *schit*, Germ, *scheit*, shingle, a piece of wood split thin, a billet. Cf. Boss-Toll. For the power of the tongue as the organ of expression of the thoughts and desires of the mind, cf. Thos. Ercel. 688.

[1] So in the Latin, cf. Blümmner, *op. cit.* pp. 6, 24, 35; in the O. Fr., cf. Voigt, *op. cit.* p. 13; Gautier, *op. cit.* pp. 375-6. For the German, cf. Schultz, *op. cit.* i. p. 215; Wackernagel, *op. cit.* p. 155, note 2, etc. Comp. "the teeth in her head . . . shone like pearls," Leahy i. pp. 13, 92; ii. p. 155; vi. p. 100. Cf. Willms, *op. cit.* p. 21; Sec. Sec. p. 69.

tiful teeth are described as a mark of feminine loveliness.[2]   Of
Eve it is said, *os ornat eburneus ordo . . . dens ebur,* Gir.
Cam. I. 349.   Likewise, of a charming daughter of Eve we are
told,

> hire teth aren white ase bon of whal,
> euene set ant atled al,   Bödd. W. L. v. 40;
> Vche tooþ as Iuory,   Cur. Mun. 9359 (Cf. Bev. O. 401).

Helen has not only white teeth, but the gums are of such fair
redness that the two colors are like the rose and the lily;

> To telle of hire tethe þat tryetly were set,
> Alse qwyte & qwem as any qwalle bon,
> Wele cumpast in cours & clenly to gedur,
> By rule in þe rede gomys as a rose faire,
> þat with lefes of þe lylly were lappit by twene,   Dest. Tr.[3] 3054.

Once a Saracen's head is described, and among the items mentioned are " whyte teeth " (Rich. 3188); he is otherwise black.

The descriptions of ugly teeth are entirely conventional.
They must be hard (Grail. 38. 410), black or yellow, and as
long and strong as boar's tusks.[4]   Of the Devil it is said " ant

---

[2] But Lydgate describes Mercury with,

> Hys tethe eke white as evory,
> Wel set in ordre by and by,   Reson and Sens. 1717.

Cf. also Chaucer, Rom. Rose, 2280, 3747 where the white teeth of men are
appreciated.

[3] The description is beautiful, but the old Scotchman is merely following his Latin original, cf. Guido, sig. d$_4$ recto 2.

[4] So in the Latin, cf. Blümmner, *op. cit.* pp. 43, 75, 69, 132; in the O. Fr.
cf. Voigt, *op. cit.* p. 60; Loubier, *op. cit.* p. 94; Schultz, *op. cit.* I. 221.   Cf.
also Kölbing's note to Ipom. 6150. Comp. Child, *op. cit.* II. 302, St. 10; II.
302, St. 7; Mabinog. " her teeth were long and yellow, more yellow were
they than the flower of the broom," p. 209.   Comp. also Chaucer's, " Gat-
tothed was she," C. T., A. 468, and cf. Skeat's note, vol. v. p. 44.   Wohlgemuth, *op. cit.* p. 31, finds that in color the teeth of French giants are
"glänzend weiss"; but Voigt, *op. cit.* p. 60, notes that this occurs in descriptions of men who are white in only two places, namely, in the teeth
and eyes.   Cf. also Geissler, *op. cit.* pp. 54 f.   That the teeth of giants
are strong as those of wild animals is suggested by the fact that they often
kill their enemies with their teeth (cf. Ferum. 3190 and note); or they
eat whole bulls at a meal (cf. Oct. S. 927; Lib. Des. 844; Laȝ. 25679;
Cur. Mun. 7453; R. Glouc. 4212; comp. Alis. L. 6126), or devour several

his grisliche teeð semden of swart irn," Marh. fol. 44, a2 (Cf. Willms, *op. cit.* p. 21 for other citations). Certain cannibal peoples have teeth as " yolowe as wax " (Alis. L. 6122), and others are so black that even their teeth are " noo white to see " (Gener. 1942). Hideous giants are generally fitted out with boar's teeth (cf. Alis. L. 6123, 6816 Oct. S. 929; Iwein. 262; Mort. Arth. 1075; Ipom. A. 6150; Sow. Bab. 2197; Alis. C. 609 and note), and the mermaids whom Alexander meets are " as biche sons tothed " (Alis. C. 5482). I have found only one description of the teeth of an ugly woman; namely, of the foul and loathly Dame Ragnell;

> She had two tethe on euery syde,
> As borys tuskes, I wolle nott hyde,
> Of lengthe a large handfulle,
> The one tusk went up and the other down,   Wed. Gaw. 549.

§ 9.   VOICE.

Angels, other heavenly visitors, and martyred saints always speak with soft voices and sweet, mild and clear;

> þo cam a swete voiz a-doun fram heuene,   Horst. D. 48. 130.

Cf. further ' swet stevin,' Sc. Leg. 1. 15; v. 573; 17. 144; 25. 452, 1566; 20. 265, 325; 38. 327; ' Jesu Criste with mylde steuen,' Seg. Mely. 68, 113; Rich. 6888; Rol. & Vern. 150; Sc. Leg. 27. 1556; 28. 282; Sev. Sag. 3836; Boc. x. 426; ' clere stewyne,' Sc. Leg. 3. 771; 19. 57. Christian men under torture sing with " hey voice & clere " (Sc. Leg. 31. 110; 36. 292), or they speak with ' blyth stewyne,' Sc. Leg. 26. 488.

The voices of women should be pleasant to hear, soft, flexible, sweeter than the music of harp or psaltry, and their speech more

---

children with ease (Mort. Arth. 1024, 1088). They go into battle with much gnashing of teeth (cf. Mort. Arth. 1076, Trev. VII. 377; I. 159; Alis. C. 5321; Laȝ. 1887), so that the foam flies out of their mouths in a most horrible manner (cf. Ferum. 698, 3888; R. Glouc. 4233. Bev. O. 3593 and note; Dest. Tr. 1957).

precious than pearls or spices (cf. Lob. Frau. 64 ff.; Bödd. W.
L. v. 30). Of Eve it is said,

> Vox dulcis, vox flexibilis, jocunda, sonora,
> Gratia cantandi non mediocris adest (Gir. Cam. I. 350),

and of Queen Olympias we are told that

> Seilde scheo spak, and nought loude,
> As wimmen that beon proude, Alis. L. 283.

Cf. further 'sche is softe of speche,' Gower, v. 2478; Rol. &
Vern. 867; Lob. Frau. 45. This gentleness and softness of
women's voices is sometimes likened to that of angels (cf. Erl.
Tol. 352; Boc. 8. 1269).

On the other hand, men should have loud, fierce voices sounding in the clamour of battle like the blast of a trumpet or the roar
of a lion.[1]   Arthur has a voice " kenliche & lude, swa bicumeð
kinge," (Laȝ. 20648); Priam has a " furse steuyn " (Dest. Tr.
3665; cf. Gir. Cam. v. 238); of Alexander it is said,

> His steuyn stiffe was & steryn þat stonayd many,
> And as a lyon he lete quen he loude romys (Alis. C. 611),

and the voice of St. Bartholomew *quasi tuba vehemens est* (Gir.
Cam. II. 69; comp. Chaucer, C. T., A. 2174).

Various historical characters are described as follows; *voce
quassa* (Gir. Cam. v. 303, cf. Conq. Ire. ' grete speche,' p. 88;
Higd. VIII. 393, cf. ' dym voys,' Trev.); *voce exili* (Gir. Cam.
v. 272, cf. Conq. Ire. p. 54, 'sproty, small spech'); *ex parvo
frigore cito raucus,* Joc. Brak. 29. Demosthenes is said to have
had a " well smal voys " (Trev. III. 330), with which we may
compare Chaucer's Pardoner whose voice is " as smal as hath a
goot" (C. T., A. 688), and the more appreciative description,
"his vois gentil & smal " (*ibid.* 3360).

Lisping, stuttering, and stammering are mentioned in con-
nection with great characters, but nowhere with disapproval.
William Rufus has a hesitancy of speech especially when angry
(R. Glouc. 8572; Wm. Malms. 504); Hector is said to have

---

[1] Comp. Philos. 2556; Sec. Sec. 116, "He þat hauys a greet voys, and
well sownand, shal be a fyghter, and wel-spekand."

" stotid " a little (Dest. Tr. 3881) ; and Neoptholomus also
" stutid full stithly, þat stynt hym to speke " (Dest. Tr. 3825;
Lyd. II. 4648; cf. Guido, *in loquela balbutiens,* sig. e₂ recto 1).
The Douglas is said to have lisped somewhat, but it became him
wonderfully well (Barb. I. 393). This need count nothing
against his prowess, however, because Hector was a great man
" And wlipsyt alsua " (*ibid.* I. 399). Chaucer's Frere also
has a very becoming lisp,

> Somwhat he lipsed, for his wantonesse,
> To make his English swete up-on his tonge, C. T., A. 264.

Eloquence of speech is spoken of in terms of the highest
praise. St. Magdalene is greatly loved " for þe swetenesse eek
of hyr eloquency, Wych from hyr mouth cam so plesauntly "
(Boc. 8. 810), and Ulysses is of all people " in his tyme most
elloquent " (Lyd. II. 4606; Dest. Tr. 3792; cf. further Dest.
Tr. 3748; Lyd. II. 4540, 4578). One very terrible voice is
described as resembling the bellow of a bull,

> He was rughher than any ku,
> And spaak als an helle bu (Alis. L. 5956),

and a subdued devil speaks in a " sneuelyng voys," Boc. I. 482

§ 10. CHIN.

A lovely chin is said to be ' choice ' and to accord well with
beautiful cheeks and face. Of Eve it is said,

> *Terminus inferior capitis producitur apte*
> *Mentum, comcludens omnia fine bono,* Gir. Cam. I. 349.

Cf. further ' hire chyn ys chosen,' Bödd. W. L. v. 34; ' chinne
choice to beholde,' Alis. A. 183; ' Lufflye of chynne and
cheke,' Ipom. 2374; ' Hir chin accordeth to the face,' Gower,
VI. 775. One infatuated lover chooses the cheek and chin of
his beloved in preference to a carbuncle (Bödd. W. L. I. 10);
the fair Egare " berys þe whyte chynne " (Emar. 924) ; and
Sir Gawain's temptress is described, " Wyth chynne & cheke ful

swete (Gaw. & Gr. Kn. 1204). A small dimple greatly adds to the beauty of the chin.[1] Of Helen it is said that

> Hir chyn full choice was the chekys benethe,
> With a dympull full derne, daynté to se (Dest. Tr. 3059),

and the chin of St. Margaret, which is as plain and smooth as polished marble, is " clouyn in tweyne " (Boc. I. 212).

Since the chins of men are generally covered with beard, any direct reference to the chin is probably a reference to the beard.[2] Thus the Christ is said to have received blows on the " softe chin " (Cur. Mun. 25490), and it is further stated that " Forked feire þe chyn he bere (Cur. Mun. 18843; cf. Trist. 686).

The chin bent back, receding, or touching on the breast is exceedingly ugly.[3] The terrible Geoffrey, Archb. of York, is described with *mento reflexo, simulantoque risui . . . valde accommodo* (Gir. Cam. IV. 420), and of the forest giant it is said that, " His chin was fast until his brest," Iw. & Gaw. 265. The old hag who accompanies Sir Gawain's beautiful temptress has a " blake chyn," Gaw. & Gr. Kn. 957.

§ 11. FACE, COUNTENANCE.

The face of a beautiful woman should be well-formed (*tretis*), not too lean, showing good breeding (*gentle*), sweet and fair. Cf. ' vysage . . . fair & treyts,' Ferum. 5883 (cf. note) ; ' face feir to fonde.' Bödd. W. L. x. 15 ; Boc. 6. 84 ; ' hir face beuteuous,' Boc. x, 386 ; IX. 552 ; ' gentle viis, bi godes sond,' Arth. & Merl. 744 ; Alis. L. 168. Speaking of women in gen-

---

[1] So also in the French (cf. Loubier, *op. cit.* p. 95), and in the German especially, cf. Schultz, *op. cit.* I. 215 ; Weinhold, DF. I. 226. Weinhold says further that the chin must be round, and as white as ivory or as snow or as the lily, *ibid.*, p. 226.

[2] But cf. Sec. Sec. p. 229, " Tho men wyche haue grete chynnes bene stronge and hardy . . . And tho that haue the chynne smale and febille bene nesshe."

[3] So in other languages, cf. Loubier, *op. cit.* p. 96 ; Wohlgemuth, *op. cit.* 28.

eral, the poet says that no man can write with ink the " swet-nesse þat þai han in face," Lob. Frau. 146. Of certain maidens held in bondage and made to work and starve it is said that their " face war lene and als unclene," Iw. & Gaw. 2971; cf. Horst. A. 3. 23; Gower, VIII. 2829.

The features of fair ladies are always regular, faultless and well-formed. Cf. 'fautles of hir fetures,' Gad. & Gr. Kn. 1760; 'þe fairest of ffeturs þat euer on fote yode,' Dest. Tr. 1018, 3019, 4001, 1307, 13182, 9132.

As for a man, his face must be long and broad (but not too much so), strong and well-formed, with features fair and just rightly made. The Abbot Samson is fine looking, *vultum habens nec rotundum nec oblongum* (Joc. Brak. 29); the Christ has a " visage lange but dele " (Sc. Leg. XI. 92); the bold Golagrus is described "With vesage lufly and lang (Goll. & Gaw. 88); and Thos. Randolph " With braid visage, plesand and fair," Barb. x. 280. Comp. Gir. Cam. VIII. 279; Trev. VI. 253; Horst. D. 27. 1183. Cf. further ' faire visage,' Cur. Mun. 18857; R. Brunn. 3137; 'grete face,' Dest. Tr. 1250; 'straught vysage,' Troy H. 1084; ' stronge vysage,' Guy B. 7408; 'brode face,' Dest. Tr. 3848; Guy B. 4289; ' angelik of visage,' Horst. C. Misc. 20a. 343; ' His face es fair withouten threpe,' Horst. C. 24. 87. Giraldus mentions a custom of the English people, not known among the Irish, of artificially elongating the face, *non enim obstetrices aquae calentis beneficio . . . faciem deprimunt,* Gir. Cam. v. 150. Of the features of the Green Knight it is said, " alle his fetures folʒande . . . ful clene " (Gaw. & Gr. Kn. 145; cf. 866), and Jason's " face was fresshe to behold And all ffetures to ffynd fourmed o right," Dest. Tr. 458 (cf. *ibid.* 129, 2865). The English youths in the Roman slave market are *lineamentorum gratia* (Wm. Malms. 63; R. Brunn. 7312).

This beauty of face and features is sometimes expressed by the alliterative combinations; [1]

---

[1] There are other combinations with *fair* (used almost innumerable times but without any definite meaning), which may be mentioned here; ' Fair

(a), *Fair of face.* 'Scho . . . watȝ so fayr of face,' Gaw. & Gr. Kn. 1259. Cf. further *ibid.* 103; Cur. Mun. 4263; Ipom. 2075, 2692; Alis. L. 4988; Alis. C. 5476; Horst. C. Misc. 23. 32; Horst. B. Misc. 5. 52, 352; Seg. Mely. 844; Rol. & Vern. 614; Oct. S. 1165; Lyd. ii. 4654; Boc. 7. 19; 9. 68; 2. 701; 6. 132; Bon. Flor. 566; Eger. & Gr. 6, 840, 1460; Sow. Bab. 226; Horst. D. 225; Grail. 32. 20.

(b), *Fair of facioun.* 'That lady fayre of facyown,' Ipom. A. 111, 7604; Cur. Mun. 22322: Lib. Des. 513, 600, 836; Sc. Leg. 30. 49; 31. 62.

A very large, long, broad, and flat face is considered loathly and grisly.[2] Cf. 'loþly was his visage made,' Cur. Mun. 7447; Gener. 2152; Alis. L. 5601, 5660; 'þe face gretly rlak, for it wes awful & mysmade' (Devil), Sc. Leg. 9. 216; Horst. 55. 177; 'þe grete visage' (giant), Bev. A. 2585; Guy. C. 7590; 'face . . . ful brade and flat' (giant), Iw. & Gaw. 259; 'Betwene hys foretop and hys chyn Length of an elle' (giant), Oct. S. 933; Alis. L. 6446; 'four fet in þe face' (Vernagu), Rol. & Ot. 476; 'his visage was both great & grim' (dwarf), Degree P. 646; Alis. L. 6424, 6414; *facie canina* Gir. Cam. iv. 420; *facie feminea, ibid.* v. 272; *facie macilenta,* Hen. Hunt. 87.

Wrinkles, scars, pimples caused by too much drinking or eating, freckles, and whelks of all kinds are marks of ugliness. Cf. *Crispatur cutis in rugas,* Gir. Cam. i. 354; 'thi vesage es crounkilde & waxen olde' (taunt to Charles), Rol. Ot. 1252; Gaw. & Gr. Kn. 952; Gower, i. 1683; *vir subrufus, lentiginosus,* Gir. Cam. v. 272 (cf. Conq. Ire. 54, 'he was samroed'). Henry II. is spoken of as a *vir subrufus, caesius* (Gir. Cam. v. 303), to which a note says, *caesii dicuntur Lintiginosi, quia caesam faciem habere vedentur.* According to Guido the King of Persia has *faciem lentiginosam* (*op. cit.* sig. e$_2$ verso 2), but

as flower in field,' Bödd. W. L. x. 26, etc.; 'feyr on hewe,' Dest. Tr. 3061, etc.; 'feyre and clere,' Bon. Flor. 1565; 'feir and shene,' Horst. C. i. 123; 'faire & briȝt,' Cur. Mun. 7885, etc.

[2] Comp. Chaucer, "Rounde was his face," C. T., A. 3934; Mabinog. "High cheeks had she, and a face lengthened downwards" (ugly black maiden), p. 209; Sec. Sec. pp. 115, 228; Philos. 2640 ff.

Lydgate, not understanding the word, says that he " had wertis plente in his face " (Lyd. ii. 4773), and the author of Dest. Tr. translates, " fellest of colour" (Dest. Tr. 3856). Likewise Cassandra is wonderfully beautiful except that in her face in sundry places there are " Many wertys growyng here & þere " (Lyd. ii. 5001), which is again a misunderstanding of Guido's description, *lentiginosa facie* (sig. e₂ recto 1). The author of Dest. Tr. also does not get the real meaning of Guido whom he renders " waike of hir colour " (Dest. Tr. 3994).³ Polidarius, the hard drinker and high liver, is " pluccid as a porke fat " (Dest. Tr. 3837) ; a foul leper is described with " pokkys and bleynes bloo " (Bon. Flor. 2023) ; and Chaucer's Somnour with his " fyr-reed cherubinnes face " is in the worst condition of all,

> For sawcefleem he was . . . .
> Ne oynement that wolde clense and byte,
> That him might helpen of his whelkes whyte,
> Nor of the knobbes sitting on his chekes,   C. T., A. 625 ff.

One of Chaucer's noble warriors, however, has

> A fewe fraknes in his face y-spreynd,
> Bitwixen yelow and somdel blak y-meynd   (C. T., A. 2167),

which does not appear to be in any way against his good appearance.

It seems that scars received in battle enhance the beauty of noble knights, being a mark of valour. Laudine loves Yvain

> For in hys face sho saw a wounde   (Iw. & Gaw. 1720)

and of a valiant French knight it is said that his face was so cut up by swords " That it our till neir wemmyt wass " (Barb. xx. 367). He expresses his wonder that the face of so good a warrior as the Douglas is unscarred but receives the answer, " love god, all tym had I Handis myne hede for till were " (*ibid.* 378). Regarding the mark between the eyebrows of Helen, Lydgate is

---

³ This process of defaming the fair Cassandra begins with Benoit,

> Rose et la cheire e lentillose   (Roman de Troie, 5511).

His source merely states, *ore. rotundo, rufam*, Dares, cap. xii.

very careful to let it be known that it is Guido and Dares who consider it an embellishment. Guido thinks she was beautiful,

> Saue he seide, in a litel space,
> A strype þer was endlonge hir face,
> Whiche, as he writ, becam hir wonder wel,
> Embelyssching hir beute euerydel,
> Like as Dares [4] makeþ discripcioun,   Lyd. II. 4527.

Countenance. The countenance of a beautiful woman should be frank and open, ' goodly,' ' lossum,' ' pleasant,' ' lovely,' and ' simple.' Cf. *frons libera,* Gir. Cam. I. 349 ;, ' lossum chere,' Bödd. W. L. II. 15 ; Iw. & Gaw. 214 ; ' luffly of lere,' Dest. Tr. 398 ; Erl. Tol. 366 ; ' countenance plesand,' Sc. Leg. 16. 227 ; Boc. 8. 803 ; ' chere . . . goodly,' Gener. 146 ; ' semblant soft and stabile,' Iw. & Gaw. 210 ; ' simpil chere,' Sev. Sag. 3578 ; Amad. 411. Bishop Baldwin also is *vultu simplici ac venusto* (Gir. Cam. VI. 148), and William II. *fronte fenestra* (Wm. Malms. 504 ; R. Brunn. 10421).

As expressing the inward emotions of gladness, joy, sorrow, and anger the countenance is often described. Cf. *vultu . . . hilari ac sereno,* Gir. Cam. v. 323 (comp. Conq. Ire. p. 98, ' glad semblant ') ; Guy. A. 7303 ; Sev. Sag. 404, 710 ;, Sec. Leg. 20. 91 ; 26. 979 ; 31. 25 ; Gower, VI. 707 ; VII. 4798 ; Boc. 9. 634 ; Horst. D. 47. 92 ; ' gladsum chere,' Sc. Leg. 3. 632 ; ' blyþe cher,' Guy A. 5632 ; ' light cher,' Iw. & Gaw. 1116 ; ' chere demure,' Boc. 5. 40 ;, ' gud chere,' Sc. Leg. 22. 485 ; ' myld chere,' Boc. 9. 634 ; ' debonayr chere,' Boc. III. 115 ; ' sorrowful chere,' Sc. Leg. 16. 468 ; ' sad cher,' Boc. II. 115 ; ' drery chere,' Sc. Leg. 22. 614 ; ' hevy cheired,' Gower, VIII. 2533 ; ' Sobyr cher,' Sc. Leg. 3. 484 ; ' wroth chere,' Sev. Sag. 2725 ; ' lourand chere,' Buy A. St. 95. 9 ; ' foule . . . of chere,' Bev. A. 2504 ;, ' chere grynyng,' Boc. 3. 898 ; ' crabbit counten-

---

[4] As a matter of fact Dares does not mention the embellishing quality of the mark at all ; he merely says, *notam inter duo supercilia habentem,* cap. XII. It is Benoit who feels that the bald statement should be qualified,

> Aveit un seing en tel endreit,
> Que merveilles li avenit   (Roman de Troie, 5135),

and Guido and the others follow him.

ance,' Sc. Leg. 37. 199; 'Malencolius of face, look and cheer,'
Horst. C. Misc. 20b. 464. Both Frederick I. and Marcus Au-
relius are said to have had stolid countenances which changed
neither in joy or sorrow, nor in anger (cf. Gir. Cam. VIII. 280;
Hen. Hunt. 25). But the ideal hero has a fierce, stern countenance, especially in battle. Cf. *facie fera,* Wm. Malms. 458;
vultu acerrimo, Gir. Cam. v. 234 (cf. Conq. Ire. p. 99, ' sterne
semblant '; 'rude sembland,' Iw. & Gaw. 629; ' sturne vysage,'
Ferum. 3401; ' stur chere,' Sc. Leg. 20. 649; 'surdy chere,'
Boc. 10. 612; ' a loke þat was laithe like out of wit,' Dest. Tr.
3797; ' Face fell as þe fyre,' Gaw. & Gr. Kn. 847. King Richard is so fierce in battle that

> Whoso hadde sene hys cuntenaunce,
> Wolde euer had hym in remembraunce, Rich. 6925.

Only the good King Priam "Was of his chere benigne and
gracious," Lyd. II. 4780.

Showing power, majesty, holiness, and bliss, the countenances of angels and redeemed saints are gloriously radiant,
shining like the sun at midday or like the fire. Under deep
spiritual excitement the faces of holy men are transfigured thru
spiritual exaltation until they resemble those of angels in brightness. An angel is " so faire and briȝt " that his appearance is
" as is þe rede lempninge " (Cur. Mun. p. 986. 107) or "like to
the fire " (*ibid.* 17372); from the face of the Christ there comes
such a gleam that it is " as It had bene a sonebeme " (Sc. Leg.
25. 445); St. Magdalene appears in a vision with " visage as
bles of fyre " (Sc. Leg. 16. 296; Boc. 8. 852), and when she
later appears before her Bishop, she is so bright that " he no
mocht behald hyre face." (Sc. Leg. 16. 936; Horst. C. 6. 234;
Boc. XIII. 79; Marh. fol. 40 a2 and note). The transfigured
face of the Christ was brighter than the sun (Sc. Leg. 1. 637),
so that when a great painter came to make his picture he could
not bear to look him in the face because of the radiance of it
(Sc. Leg. XI. 72). St. Machor " schane of halyness " (Sc. Leg.
27. 318), or to be more exact " schenis as a ȝeme " (*ibid.* 380),
and when St. Stephen is being stoned his face shines as though

it were an angel's (Horst. C. 6. 99).   Comp. Cur. Mun. 19417;
R. Brunn. 14918; Horst. D. 7. 68; 29. 26; 40. 171; 42. 182;
66. 724; 73. 159; Cur. Mun. 18831).

§ 12.   SKIN, SKIN OF FACE.

The skin of beautiful women and children must be smooth,
flawless, soft as silk, and above all shining white.[1]   Cf. ' þi
skyne þat is so nessche,' Horst. C. Misc. 21. 416; ' hir body softe
as silke,' Horst. C. p. 238. 209; ' faire of skin,' Horst. C. 33.
25; Horn. 1015; ' tender of skinne,' Alis. A. 194; ' þi white
flesche,' Horst. C. Misc. 3. 132, 144; 5. 176; p. 496. 239; p.
493. 138; ' Hire flesche þat was so white and shene,' Horst. B.
Misc. 6. 226.

The adjective *white* is very commonly used to describe beautiful women and children and handsome men as well.   The
word is synonymous, for the most part, with beautiful,[2] and
when used alone, is probably meant to describe the skin in
general.   Definite descriptions of the whiteness of the skin are
also to be found here.   Cf. *Erat . . . vir albus,* Gir. Cam. v.
344 (cf. Conq. Ire. 118); *caro candida, ibid.* II. 68; ' white &
clere,' R. Brunn. 14880, 14889; ' quite hide,' Cur. Mun. 28016,
9120; Pier. Lang. 956; Alis. L. 4163; Orf. 97; Gower, v.
2469; Lyd. II. 5000; ' lemman white & fre,' Rol. & Ot. 1324;
' wayle whyte,' Bödd. W. L. VII. 60; ' fayre and white,' Thos.

---

[1] So in the Latin, cf. Blümmner, *op. cit.* p. 4, 19, 40; in the Old French,
cf. Loubier, *op. cit.* pp. 70, 114; Ott, *op. cit.* p. 90; in the German, cf.
Weinhold DF. p. 226; Wackernagel, *op. cit.* p. 161; in the Old Norse, cf.
Weinhold AL. 31.   In Old Eng. *whīt,* when applied to angels who live in
the light of heaven, is largely symbolic, cf. Mead, *P. M. L. A.* 14. pp. 179,
180, n. 1.   In descriptions of allegorical figures " gilt Weiss . . . als
diejenige Farbenbenennung, welche das Gute und Schöne kennzeichnet,"
cf. Willms, *op. cit.* p. 26, 20-25.   Comp. Leahy, I. 94; II. 37, 155.   One of
the tokens of a good complexion is " a tendyr skynne," Sec. Sec. p. 223.

[2] So in the German, " schön ist im Deutschen von je her ein gleichbe-
deutendes Wort mit *weiss* gewesen, wie . . . im Griechischen und im
Serbischen *weiss* zugleich den Sinn von schön besizt," Wackernagel, *op.
cit.* I. 161, 163.   Cf. Kaluza to Lib. Des. 850 and Intro. CIV.

Ercel. L. 239; Dest. Tr. 3742, 3994; Trev. I. 53, 267; R. Glouc. 565, 182; Horst. D. 25. 50; 45. 676; 62; 63; 'þi bodi is white,' Gregor. A. 855; Orph. 103, 'Faire and whyte is hire face,' Alis. L. 7587, 6053; Gregor. C. 853; *ibid.* v. 1025; *ibid.* R. 423; Horst. D. 27. 2175; Guy. A. 4884; Guy. B. 941; 'whyte lere,' Gowth. 61; Horst. C. Misc. 22. 138.

Among the many beautiful comparisons used to give some idea of the splendid whiteness of the skin are;

(a), *White as whale's bone,* i. e. as white as ivory, the bone or tooth of the walrus (cf. Herrtage to Ferum. 2429). The comparison occurs only in descriptions of feminine loveliness. Cf. 'His wyfe es whitte as walles bone,' Isum. C. 250; Emar. 33; Ferum. 2429; Bödd. W. L. VII. 1; Thos. Ercel. L. 235, 239; Horst. C. Misc. 4. 281; Degree P. 16; Torr. 794; Squyr. 71; Parton, Frag. 17.

(b), *White as the sea foam.*[3] Cf. 'Hir lyre es als þe sea fome,' Isum. C. 250; Emar. 497, 818; Torr. 31; Rol. & Ot. 967; Sc. Leg. 24. 104.

(c), *White as milk or as the foam of milk.*[4] This comparison is used only in descriptions of women and youths. Cf. 'A lady . . . white so mylk,' Iw. & Gaw. 819; Horst. D. 59. 321; Gregor. V. 807; Horn. Ch. 295; Sc. Leg. 9. 50; 28. 23; Adler, 7. 13; Dest. Tr. 3985; 'Hyr skyn as whyt so þe melke fom,' Ferum. 5879; 'Melk white was her face,' Lib. Des. 944; Troy. H. 1338.

(d), *White as chalk.* Cf. 'The childire ware chalke-whitte chekys and oþer,' Mort. Arth. 3329; 'a chalke-whitte maydene,' Dest. Tr. 3047.

(e), *White as swan or as feather of swan.*[5] Cf. 'Iosyan, That was whyte as any swan,' Bev. O. 3601; Lib. Des. 1456; Torr. 759; Le Mort. Arth. 1141; Sow. Bab. 2749; Max. 157;

---

[3] Cf. Kölbing to Ipom. 2384; Lüdtke to Erl. Tol. 199.
[4] Cf. Kaluza to Lib. Des. 132; Lüdtke to Erl. Tol. 199; Kölbing to Ipom. 2384; Zielke to Orf. p. 19; *Anglia*, 28. p. 39; *ibid.*, 27. p. 576; *ibid.*, I. p. 213; Kläber, Das Bild bei Chaucer, pp. 49. 10.
[5] For other citations cf. Willms, *op. cit.* p. 29; Kaluza to Lib. Des. 1457; Lüdtke to Erl. Tol. 199.

This. Ercel. C. 68; ' As white as feþer of swan,' Tars. 11;
Horn. Ch. 76; Horst. B. 5. 45; Gregor. v. 203; ' The third
maister was litel man, Faire of chere and white as swan,' Sev.
Sag. 77; ' Two man chylderyn . . . As whytte as swan,' Oct.
S. 101.

(f), *White as flower,*[6] *or as the blossom on briar, or as thẹ́
lily flower.*   This comparison is used generally in descriptions
of fair maidens and beautiful youths.   Cf. ' lady white so
flowre,' Sev. Sag. 2956; Horn. 14; Rich. 138; Launf. M. 260,
387; Launf. R. 69, 105; Iw. & Gaw. 1421; Oct. S. 40; Gowth.
377; ' Whyte sche was as felde flowre,' Emar. 729; Troy H.
1572; Bon. Flor. 194, 1343, 2050; Kn. of Cour. 97; ' As whyt
as blosme on tre,' Isum. 252 (cf. Willms, *op. cit.* p. 28) ; ' Sche
was whyte as blossme on flowre,' Triam. C. 628.   Closely related to this ' white as a blossom ' is the comparison ' *bright* as
a blossom,' where bright means " blendendes weiss " according
to Willms (cf. *op. cit.* p. 26).   Cf. ' Brihtest bleo of alle þat
euer iboren weren, blosme iblowen ' (Christ), Marh. fol. 45.
b6; Oct. N. 40; Athel. 72; ' As bryȝt as blosme on bowȝ,' Athel.
290; Bödd. W. L. i. 17; ' A maide . . . as briȝt as blosme on
brere,' Lib. Des. 624; Launf. M. 934; Launf. R. 428; Erl.
Tol. 332; Horst. C. Misc. 11. 213, 524; Gregor. R. 47; *ibid.*
V. 286, 431, 331; *ibid.* A. 773, 721, 165, 57; ' þat lady bryȝt so
blosme on þe brom,' Gregor. R. 298; ' Doghtur bryght as blome,'
Bon. Flor. 686; Le Mort. Arth. 724, 835; Gregor. V. 203.

As white as the lily flower is an especially beloved comparison.   Cf. ' Also whyt as lylye-flour ' (children), Athel. 70;
' She was white as lely in May,' Launf. R. 103; Le Mort. Arth.
2994; Eglam. 145; Emar. 66, 205; Gowth. B. 373; Bon. Flor.
901, 1023, 1539; Triam. P. 649; Iw. & Gaw. 2510; Guy B.
4754; Torr. 1639; Isum. E. 251; Parton. Frag. 39, 67, 83;
' Liliwhite was hur liche to likne þe beurde,' Alis. A. 195;
Cur. Mon. 25629; Bödd. W. L. i. 12; *ibid.* ix. 46; Pist. Sus.
16; Oct. N. 1363; Launf. M. 292.

---

[6] Cf. Kaluza to Lib. Des. 1489; Zupitza to Athel. 70 & 72; Lüdtke to
Erl. Tol. 200; Zielke to Orf. pp. 9, 19; and Willms, *op. cit.* p. 28 for other
citations and further discussion.

(g), *As white or bright as a ray of the sun, or as starlight, or as a lantern.* Cf. ' Whit so eny sonne,' Horn. 691; 'ladi briht so day,' Gregor. V. 289; Bödd. W. L. xi. 2; 'Briht so sonne on Rouwel bon,' *ibid.* 1268; ' Bryght as the sonne thorugh glas,' Rich. 75; Ipom. 5020 and note; Thos. Ercel. T. 47; ' Ase sonnebem hire bleo ys briht,' Bödd. W. L. v. 7; Alis. L. 281; ' Myn neb þat wes so bryht So eny sterre lyht,' Max. 226; Trist. 2971; ' briʒtere þan ani gold ' [7] Horst. A. 4c. 505; Bödd. W. L. vi. 3; x. 23; Gir. Cam. i. 353; ' briʒt so beiʒe,' Trist. 2171, 3162; Horst. A. 4c. 502; 'Briʒter þan þe rouwel bon,' Gregor. V. 1268. Angels and transfigured martyrs are said to shine like the sun, or like the daylight, or like a gleam. The redeemed in heaven " shalt be briʒte as sonne þan; shal be briʒtere . . . Seuen siþe þen sonne now," Cur. Mun. 23393; Boc. 3. 811; 8. 1286; Sc. Leg. 30. 735; 4. 294; Alis. L. 7511; ' Bryʒtere þan any leme,' Horst. D. 14. 70; Horst. C. Misc. 3. 65, 134; *ibid.* p. 491, 53; *ibid.* p. 494, 164.

(h), *As white or bright as the glass,*[8] *or as ivory*—applied mostly in descriptions of women and youths. Cf. ' Sabren hit highte, as white as glas,' R. Brunn. 2081. This doubtless refers to the skin, glossy, and as glancing and glistening as glass. Comp. Horn. 14; Pier. Lang. 2318; Guy. A. 131. Willms produces one other quotation where the description runs, " Hyr vysayge whyt as playn yuore," Pearl, 178.

(i), *As white as silk, or as snow.* Cassandra is said to have been " as the silke white," Dest. Tr. 3993 (Guido, *candida multum,* sig. e₃ r. 3). In the description of Eve we are told,

> *Nuda sedet, niveusque nitor radiosus in undis*
> *Fulget, et umbrosum non sinit esse locum,* Gir. Cam. i. 352.

Cf. Gir. Cam. i. 353; ' Whyt as snow on downe,' Launf. M. 241; ' (White as) snow þat sneweþ on winteres day' Launf. M. 292; Launf. R. 103; Horst. B. 2. 536; Alis. C. 5482; 'hude

---

[7] Comp. Chaucer,

> Ful brighter was the shyning of hir hewe,
> Than in the tour the noble y-forged newe, C. T., A. 3255, 377.

[8] Comp. Chaucer, C. T., A. 199.

snaw hwit,' Marh. fol. 51. Geoffrey of Monmouth has already exhausted almost the whole list of comparisons [9] in his description of that fair lady, Estrides; *candorem carnis ejus nec nitidum ebur, nec nix recenter cadens, nec lilia ulla vincebat,* Lib. II. Cap. 11. (For further citations cf. Willms, *op. cit.* p. 29).

As often as definite comparisons are found to aid in the delineation of the loveliness of fair women and beautiful children, the indefinite, more or less colorless epithet is far more common. In fact the general epithet is the great present aid in every time of trouble for the writers of romance and legend. It would be a useless toil to tabulate all the occurrences of those words like 'bright,' 'clere,' 'schene' etc. They are innumerable.

(a), *Bright* may at times be supposed to refer to the lustrous beauty of white skin. ' Lady bright,' even when used to fill out a line or for purposes of rime, seems to sum up all the charms of the heroine. The word is especially beloved by writers of romance, tho it is found—but much less frequently—in the legends and lyrics. It seems to have been used almost unconsciously at times; the very mentioning of the lady's name suggests 'bright'; any part of her body and all alike are 'bright'; she has bright skin, bright eyes, bright hair, bright face; and one author becomes so habituated to the use of this convenient word that he is betrayed into speaking of the " Sarʒins bryght," Torr. 2232.

(b), *Clere,* meaning brilliant, transparent, beautiful, is descriptive alike of fair women, angels, and noble knights (Cf. Ott, *op. cit.* p. 152). It is used in almost the same sense as bright, and almost as often. Occasionally it is used substantively, 'that clere' (cf. Torr. 78, 36, 1997, 2009), or in definite descriptions of skin or face. Cf. ' visage clere,' Sc. Leg. 17. 312; ' hir chekis as any cristal clere,' Lyd. IV. 589; ' cler

---

[9] Chaucer pokes fun at the romance comparisons as usual;

> Sir Thopas wex a doghty swayn,
> Whyte was his face as payndermayn,

C. T., B 1914. (Cf. Skeat's note, v. p. 184).

as the cristall,' Dest. Tr. 13182; 'cler as þe glas,' Horst. B.
Misc. 9. 42; 'coloure clere,' Kn. of Cour. 321; ' Clere of colour
so is þe wine,' Lob. Frau. 189 ; 'of vysage fayir and klere,' Parton. Frag. 56; Grail. 17. 279; 22. 333; Gregor. C. 1094;
Horst. D. 38. 132; Bödd. W. L. x. 32.

(c), *Schene,* meaning likewise beautiful, brilliant, of dazzling whiteness, holds a place of honor equal to that of bright
and clere. It occurs most often in the *caudae* of the *rime
couée* stanza. Cf. ' Blauncheflour þe schene,' Guy. A. St. 44.
97; ' Maidens shene so bon,' Max. 156.

The M. E. poets delight in emphasizing the beauty of the
person described by the use of certain formula-like combinations of common epithets. If the combinations can be made to
alliterate, they are appreciated all the more. Such combinations are:

(a), *Bright in bower*—applied always to women. Cf. ' ynot
non so freoli flour, Ase ledies þat beþ bryght in bour,' Bödd.
W. L. ix. 7; 'blisfull berde in bour,' Launf. M. 750, etc. Sometimes it is used substantively; ' þat bryꝛtt in bowr ' Gowth. A.
437; Rol. & Ot. 622, 624. The combination occurs in all eigh-
teen times.

(b), *Bright of ble*—favored especially in descriptions of
maidens and youths. Cf. ' bright of ble,' R. Brunn. 14, 913;
' douhter briꝛt on ble,' Bödd. W. L. x. 25 ; ' off ble as bryght as
sonne,' Ipom. A. 5021; ' brightest of ble,' Gol. & Gaw. 1146,
etc. etc. The combination occurs in all forty times. (Cf.
Kölbing to Ipom. 757 ; Mätzner, *bleo;* Kaluza to Lib. Des. 305 ;
Holthausen to Perc. Gal. 1829).

(c), *Bright of hew.* Cf. ' þe maiden briꝛt of hewe,' Trist.
1267; ' bryꝛt of hewe ' (young squire), Guy. B. 121; ' bryght
of hewe ' (good steward), Guy. B. 21; ' Fayr and hende and
briꝛt of hewe ' (Christ), Horst. C. Misc. 1. 179; ' glistering
hewe,' Horst. C. Misc. 24. 13; ' bryght his coloure shone,'
Ipom. A. 476. etc. Occurs thirteen times.

(d), *Bright and schene*—descriptive for the most part of
beautiful women, but it is said of the Christ that he is " bright
and schene," Cur. Mun. 25564. Cf. ' sche was briꝛt and

schene,' Trist. 1330; 'þe beurde so bryght was of ble scheene,' Alis. A. 1503; 'both bryght *and* shene,' Boc. II. 519. etc. This combination is found twenty-five times.

Brown. If a brilliant whiteness of the skin is so highly appreciated as to make white synonymous with beautiful, then a dark or brown skin should be considered ugly.[10] Indeed as Kaluza remarks (Introd. to Lib. Des. CIV), " brünett aber war gleichbedeutend mit hässlich." Libeaus and his opponent agree to place their fair ladies in the market place that bond and free may look upon them and see which is the more beautiful. Libeaus remarks,

> ȝif my lemman is broun,
> To winne þe gerfaucoun,
> Fiȝte I will wiþ þe, Lib. Des. 850 (and note).

The description of Chaucer's Dame Frauchise may be compared with this,

> She was not broun ne dun of hewe,
> But whyt as snowe y-fallen newe, Rom. Rose 1212.[11]

On the other hand, Chaucer's independent description of Curtesye must be recorded. Nothing was ever missaid of her and " Cleer broun she was " (Rom. Rose, 1262), where the original runs, *El fu clere comme la lune,* Rom. de la Rose, 1280. In general, however, a brown maid, if not absolutely ugly, is at least of low birth.

While some noble knights are said to be white, still a brown skin is highly favoured. The tenth token of a knight of

---

[10] So in the *English and Scottish Popular Ballads,* ed. Child. A brown bride is rejected because of her complexion, Vol. II. pp. 182-97. Cf. also Vol. I. 120, 133 (M10), 135 (1). For further discussion cf. Mead, W. E., Colour in the English and Scottish Popular Ballads, (in *Furnivall Miscellany*) A "nut-brown maid" seems to be the appreciated subject of many German and French folk-songs, cf. E. Flügel, *Neuenglisches Lesebuch,* p. 447; she is likewise the heroine of some of the English popular songs, cf. *ibid., loc. cit.* Cf. also Willms, *op. cit.* p. 58.

[11] Cf. corresponding Fr. original, *ne brun ne bise,* Rom. de la Rose, 1184. Comp. also Beauty, "ne she was derk ne broun, but bright, And cleer as the mone-light," Rom. Rose. 1009, with the Fr. orig. *El ne fu ascure ne brune, Ains fu clere comme la lune,* Rom. de la Rose, 1023.

" stronge Corage " is that he should be of "broune coloure in al the body," Sec. Sec. 222; 233 (Comp. Philos. p. 81. 2589). Merlin is said to have been " mickel, broun & beld " (Arth. & Merl. 1190) at the age of fifteen years; and many noble knights are called " þe broun " (cf. Arth. & Merl. 5441, 6536, 5631, 9069; ? Alis. L. 1999). While such citations may refer to the hair, they seem more likely to be descriptive of the tanned skin of knights exposed to hardships and many battles. This interpretation would explain the substantive combination, the *brown and the black*. Of one great warrior it is said that, " He felde browne, he felde blake," Havel. 2694 (Cf. further *ibid*. 2181, 2248, 2847, 1909; Pier. Lang. 4833; Am. & Am. 2473). While the combination as used here is merely one way of saying that he felled everybody in general, yet in its original significance it probably meant the bond and the free, masters and servants, the brave and the cowardly. This interpretation is suggested by the fact that in the Old Norse ' black ' is often used in the sense of ' mean,' ' low-born,' of serfs and thralls, in contrast to ' white,' meaning high-born, noble (cf. Weinhold AL. p. 33). Indeed, once in M.E. we find the substantive combination, the white and the black, which probably had originaly a like significance;

> Now haþ Charlis þe citee y-take,
> & sleyn, echon boþ whit & blake,   Ferum. 4839.

Peoples who live in hot climates are by nature brown (cf. Alis. L. 6578; Exodus, 71 ff.; comp. Mead, A. p. 193), and others who are naturally white become tanned by exposure to the sun [12] (cf. Horst. D. 39. 143).

Black. As in the descriptions of hair, *brown* may mean any dark shade of color of skin from a chestnut-brown to a decided black. If there is any doubt as to the beauty or ugliness of brown persons, it is certain that those who are black are decidedly ugly and sometimes hideous.[13] Devils, giants, and other

---

[12] Comp. Chaucer, C. T., A. 109, 394; B. 4366 for brown sunburned faces. Of Vulcan it is said that "his face was ful broune," House of Fame, 138 f.

[13] So in the Latin, cf. Blümmner, *op. cit*, pp. 40, 43, 55, 69, 97; in the O. F. cf. Loubier, *op. cit*. p. 71; Ott, *op. cit*. pp. 23, 29; in the German, cf.

children of the father Satan are black, and have hard rough
hides. Of the child Merlin, begotten of an incubus, it is said
that he " was blacker þan anoþer & wel rower " (Arth. & Merl.
980), or according to another version, " Blak he was, . . . And
rouȝh as a swyn " (cf. *ibid.* ms. L. 979; ms. D. 859). The
hide of the monster found in Mort. Arth. (1084) is " Harske as
a hunde-fisch "; and that of another loathly giant " blake and
harde," Sow. Bab. 2194 (Cf. Alis. L. 6414, 6424; Horst. D.
45. 672).

This tendency to paint everything evil, wicked, malicious,
and ugly in black colors finds full expression in descriptions of
devils.[14]   In this connection Mead supposes that the use of
black is symbolical and conventional. Cf. ' swarte deouel,'
Marh. fol. 46. b18; fol. 45; ' fendes blake,' Horst. C. 10. 77;
34. 136; Misc. 13. 388; 28. 354; Horst. D. 36. 475; 62. 205,
211; 63. 195; Sc. Leg. 20. 142; 6. 636; 25. 586. Lost souls
are black in contrast to the brightly shining souls of the redeemed. A woman who has broken her marriage vows is
" swart and swiþe ounlede," Horst. C. p. 507. 157. Cf. *ibid.*
Misc. p. 214. 119; p. 227. 132; Horst. D. 69. fol. 200 a6.
Dragons—children of the devil—are of course black. Cf.
Guy. A. 6824, 6831. (Cf. Geissler, *op. cit.* p. 60 ff.)

Certain very wicked men are also black. Cf. *colore nigeri-
mus,* Gir. Cam. iv. 420; *Si viri colorem, si vultum quaeris,
niger,* Gir. Cam. v. 354; Bishop Longis ' was bothe blak and
grysliche, And rough y-schuldreod also,' Alis. L. 6813; ' swart
ant al to swolle,' Bödd. P. L. iv. 48. Races of black men are
described, Alis. L. 5626, 6330; Trev. i. 53, 169; iv. 449;
Horst. D. 45. 686; Sc. Leg. 10. 35. St. Egipciane, after wandering in the desert, " brynt with þe sone, blak scho vas " (Sc.

Wackernagel, *op. cit.* pp. 161, 162; and in the O. Norse, cf. Weinhold AL.
p. 33. Comp. Mabinog. pp. 200, 209; Sec. Sec. p. 229. For a full discussion
of the Devil, his children, and followers, cf. Geissler, *op. cit.* pp. 48, 54;
Wohlgemuth, *op. cit.* pp. 12, 26, 38, 81.

[14] For many other citations from Anglo-Saxon and later literature, cf.
Mead A. p. 184; Willms, *op. cit.* p. 7 ff. For other lost-soul quotations cf.
Mead. A. p. 184, note 1; Willms, *op. cit.* pp. 7, 16.

Leg. 18. 23, 1007). Guy anoints himself with a black ointment so that "he was black and beschente" (Guy B. 5788).
Of Polydamus [15] we are told that his "colour blent was in
blake" (Dest. Tr. 3962).

In the romances especially we find that almost all opponents
of noble knights, and enemies to Christianity are stigmatized
as Saracens, and as such they are children and companions of
the Devil, consequently black. Cf. 'Saraȝins lodlike and
blake,' Horn. 1415; 'þe Soudan, þat was blac,' Tars. 793, 922,
445; Cur. Mun. 8077; Oct. S. 1397, 1623; Rich. 3187; Ferum.
2785; Guy. B. 3227; Guy. A. 4460; C. 7757 10321; Horst. C.
Misc. 4. 426; 6. 343. To emphasize the ugliness and wickedness of the detested enemy, various comparisons are restorted
to, the most common of which is;

(a), *As black as pitch.* Cf. 'as blak so pych' (Alagolafre),
Ferum. 4330; 'loked loþliche, & was swart as piche' (Vernagu), Rol. & Vern. 482; Guy. B. 7579; C. 7759; Lib. Des.
619, 1327, 1345; Ipom. 6156 and note; 'so blac so pych' (Saracens), Ferum, 2461; 'als blake alks pyk or lede' (burned
bodies), Horst. C. Misc. 22. 827; 'Also blak as any pycche'
(fearless man), Alis. L. 5948; 'as blak as pycche, And had a
face wel griseliche' (Old churl), Alis. L. 5599; 4913, 4972,
6416.

(b), *As black as coal or as a burned brand,* describes devils,
giants, and strange ugly peoples. Cf. ' As blac he is as brondes
brend, He semes as it were a fende, þat comen were out of helle,'
Guy. A. St. 62. 10; 'colmie snute' (Horn in disguise), Horn.
1. 161; 'A fende blacker þan any cole,' Horst. C. 24. 305;
Ferum. 2439; ' Al blak so cole-brond ' (Vetas), Alis. L. 6260;
Alis. L. 6120; Gener. 2075, 1941.

---

[15] It is somewhat surprising to find that the 'blake' color of P. is not
here considered a defect. Benôit describes him, *brun le vis,* Rom. de Troie,
5485, and Guido follows with, *Sed parum fusco colore respersus,* sig. e₂
verso 2. While Guido throws in the qualifying *sed,* still he uses the least
objectionable word at his command, *fuscus.* In Latin descriptions of
women, *niger* means a very ugly shade of black, but if the poet loves the
lady, he describes her with *fuscus* (cf. Blümmner, 98).

(c), *As black as soot,* is applied especially to devils and sometimes to giants.   Cf. ' þat ethiope as þe sete blak,' Sc. Leg. 11. 439; Sc. Leg. 9. 215; Sc. Leg. 28. 427; Ipom. 6176, ' Blakkere more than a bore '; ' blake as more (moor),' Sow. Bab. 1004; ' blak As Ony Scho,' Grail. 37. 106.

Blue.   The descriptive adjective blue, when applied to individuals or races, may mean either a very deep blue [16] or a decided black, more probably the latter.   Of the giant Beliagog we learn that he is " al blo " (Trist. 2976) which Kölbing renders " den ganz schwarzen " (p. 275).   The Saracens are said to be " Blak & blo as leed " (Cur. Mun. 8073), or of different colors, " Bloo, some yolowe, some blake as more," Tars. 1004, 1219.   Cf. ' visages ... blew so Ynde' (strange people) Alis. L. 5272 (cf. Willms, *op. cit.* p. 62) ; ' In Ynde beeþ men of colour and hewe i-died,' Trev. I. 79.   The devil is spoken of as being " muchele del blaccre þen euer ani blamon,' Marh. fol. 45 b2. Here and elsewhere there can be no doubt that ' blueman ' means negro, or a black man.   The author of Cur. Mun., speaking of Aethiopia, says, " þat londe is moost in þe souþ, þere þat blo men are ful couþ " (2117), and in a detailed description of the following of King Arthur, Laȝamon says, " Mid him com moni Aufrican, of Ethiope he brohte þa bleoman," Laȝ. 25379. Moreover, the word regularly translates Aethiopian in Trev. I. pp. 45, 157; II. pp. 9, 187, 199, 201, 285, 321, 327; VI. pp. 379. Comp. Horst. D. 55. 176.

Yellow.   Yellow skins and faces are considered exceedingly ugly [17] in descriptions of both men and women.   Of the Garra-

---

[16] For further discussion of the meaning of blue and ' bloman ' cf. Willms, *op. cit.* p. 62; and especially Cockayne to Marh. p. 97; Kölbing to Trist. (gloss). In Sec. Sec. (p. 114) we are warned to beware of men with blue skins.

[17] Comp. Chaucer, Rom. Rose, 4495, 2399, 310. Cf. Wackernagel, *op. cit.* p. 166. The citations given by Willms (*op. cit.* p. 66) from Dest. Tr. 5462, 6174 refer to the colors of a detachment of soldiers rather than to the color of their skin. The physiognomies are divided as to the significance of yellow skins. In Sec. Sec. (pp. 114, 16) we are warned against them as indicating men of wicked characters; but on p. 229 (*ibid.*) we are told, " Tho that bene yelow of coloure, bene coragious i-lyke to lyons."

nien, a people exposed to the sun, it is said that they are regular devil's sons, the foulest ' pages ' in the world and " So wex yellow is heore visages " (Alis. L. 6459), and some of the Saracens described in Sow. Bab. 1005 are also "yolowe." An ugly hag, whose duty it is to accompany and protect the beautiful white lady in Gaw. & Gr. Kn., is pictured (951) as being "ʒolʒe." (Cf. Trev. viii. p. 46).

Green and Red. The wonderful Green Knight is all over of a green hue, so that he is " enker grene," Gaw. & Gr. Kn. 147. A rough red skin is almost as ugly as a black hide. Once a loathly giant is described as having red skin (Lib. Des. 619), and the tailed mugglings, who failed to receive St. Austin well, " for þan ilke dede . . . habbeoð neb red," Laʒ. 29593.

§ 15. CHEEKS, COMPLEXION.

The cheeks of both men and women, to be beautiful, must not be pale and wan, but fresh and well-coloured.. Cf. *congruis et coloratissimus vultibus,* Gir. Cam. v. 150; *vultu colorato decentique, ibid.* v. 297 (cf. Conq. Ire. p. 303, 'vysage wel colowred becomlyche '); ' wunliche on heowen,' Laʒ. 24643; ' Of fair colour,' R. Brunn. 7599; Guy. B. 56; Alis. L. 163; Sev. Sag. 242; Gaw. & Gr. Kn. 943; ' of so fynes hewes,' *ibid.* 1761; ' semely of colowre,' Triam. C. 618; Pist. Sus. 172; ' of al farnes & coloure clere,' Sc. Leg. 30. 211; Oct. N. 1087; ' of colour neþir pale ne wan,' Boc. 5. 374; ' likyng of colour,' Dest. Tr. 3752. Freshness of colour is especially appreciated in women; " He seth hire face of such colour, That freesshere is than any flour," Gower, vi. 768. Cf. Further Boc. 9. 195, 717; 3. 33; 4. 370; Parton, 7439; Gener. 4240; Horst. D. 45. 680.

Ruddy. Such well-coloured, fresh cheeks or faces are sometimes said to be ' ruddy.' [1] Cf. ' Theo ladies schynen so the

---

[1] Comp. Chaucer, C. T., F. 385; Rom. Rose, 820; Leahy, i. pp. 13, 92; *Old English Homilies,* Vol. ii. p. 255. 13.

glas And this maidenes with rody face, Passen sone so flour on gras,' Alis. L. 7832; *ibid.* 798; Kaluza to Lib. Des. 1322; Gower, II. 385; v. 2471; Lyd. II. 4983; Troy H. 717; Conq. Ire. 54; Gir. Cam. v. 272; Conq. Ire. 98; Gir. Cam. v. 233.

The highly appreciated florid complexion of men and the rich red bloom on the cheeks of women must be carefully distinguished from the rough red skin which is so ugly. Both may be described, however, by the adjectives red or sanguine.[2]   Cf. 'His vijs somdel with reed was meynd' (Christ), Cur. Mun. 18841; 'rede man' (Wise Man), Sev. Sag. 87; 'red of face' (Charlemagne), Rol. & Vern. 434; 'Rede and fayer of flesshe and blode' (Lancelot), Le Mort. Arth. 3888; Conq. Ire. 54 (Gir. Cam. v. 272); Conq. Ire. 88 (Gir. Cam. v. 303); *colore rufo,* Wm. Malms. 504; Trev. VIII. 22; Beryn. 2132; Horst. D. 59. 182; 'reed of hew' (David), Cur. Mun. 7365; Alis. L. 7651; 'Of sangwyn hewe, havyng moche of red' (Tantalus), Lyd. II. 4560 (cf. Guido, *candidus rubore permixto,* sig. e₁ verso 2); 'rode . . . so rede' (Eurydice), Orph. 105; Orf. 97; Guy. C. 5689; Launf. M. 242; Gower, VI. 774; 'rede chekys,' Dest. Tr. 8044, 8520; 'Riche red on þat on rayled ey quere,' (young woman), Gaw. & Gr. Kn. 951.

The romances are especially rich in comparisons to express the glow and bloom on the cheeks of fair heroines and children. Such favored comparisons are;

(a) *As red as blossom on briar.* Cf. Tars. 13; Troy H. 1416; Le Mort. Arth. 179 (and note).

(b) *As red as rose* [3] *in the rain, or on the thorn, or in the*

---

[2] Comp. Chaucer, C. T., A. 2168, 3317, 333, 458; Leahy, I. 100. For a discussion of the meaning of the four complexions cf. Sec. Sec. p. 220. One of the tokens of an honest man is that he is "ruddy of colure as sanguyne." Sec. Sec. p. 223, 229. Cf. Blümmner, *op. cit.* pp. 60, 174, 186; Willms, *op. cit.* 44.

[3] Cf. also Bruce to Le Mort. Arth. 179; Zupitza to Athel. 71; Lüdtke to Erl. Tol. 200; Zielke to Orf. p. 12; Kaluza to Lib. Des. 937-8; Willms, *op. cit.* pp. 44, 49. Comp. Chaucer, C. T., A. 1038. For like comparisons in O. Fr. cf. Ott, *op. cit.* p. 104; Loubier, *op. cit.* p. 71; in the German cf. Schultz, I. 214; Weinhold, DF. i. p. 224; Wackernagel, *op. cit.* p. 209; in the Latin, cf. Blümmner, *op. cit.* p. 202; Ogle, II. p. 148.

arbor. Cf. 'Rose red was hur rode,' Alis. A. 178; Horn. 16; Bödd. W. L. I. 11; ' þe heuis swilk' in hire ler So is þe rose in roser, Hwan it is fayr sprad ut newe Ageyn þe sunne,' Havel. 2918; Gir. Cam. I. 349; Lib. Des. 937, 1322; 'clere As rose in erbere,' Lib. Des. 955; 'her rud was red as rose in raine,' Eger. & Gr. 217, 795; Launf. M. 295; R. 106; 'fresshe as rose on thorne,' Horst. B. Misc. 7. 223; Horst. C. Misc. 11. 295; Dest. Tr. 9129 3,987; Trev. VII. 266; Parton. 7399; *ibid.,* Frag. 18; Parton. R. 5157.

(c) *As red as a cherry.* Cf. 'Roddys feyre and Rede as chery,' Le Mort. Arth. 3956; 'Ye were whyte as whales bone . . . Your ruddy read as any chery,' Squyr. 711; Boc. I. 211. Chaucer gives the additional comparison, ' His rode is lyk scarlet in grayn,' C. T., B. 917 (cf. note, vol. v. 185).

(d) *White and red.* Ideally beautiful women and children, and occasionally men, are those whose complexions present an even and fair mingling of both white and red.[4] Cf. ' Wyth chynne & cheke ful swete, Boþe quit & red in-blande,' Gaw. & Gr. Kn. 1204; Horst. D. 45. 793; Bev. M. 397; Athel. 291; Eger. & Gr. 621.

(e) *White or chalk-white and rose.* Sometimes the red of such pink-and-white complexions is compared to the rose. Cf. ' eyþer cheke whit ynoh & rode on eke, ase rose when hit redes,' Bödd. W. L. v. 35; 'Hir chekes full choise, as the chalke white, As the rose was the rud þat raiked hom in,' Dest. Tr. 3047 (cf. Guido, Helen, sig. d$_4$ recto 2) ; ' Wele colouret by course, clene of his face, Rede roicond in white as the Roose fresshe ' (Tantalus), Dest. Tr. 3770 (Comp. Guido, *candidus rubore permixto,* sig. e$_1$ verso 2; and Lyd. II. 4537).

(f) *As red as blood and as white as snow,*[5] is a striking com-

---

[4] Comp. Mabinog. p. 187; Leahy, II. p. 156. One of the tokens of a perfect man is that his complexion should 'represent a mingling of white and red, cf. Sec. Sec. p. 236, 231; Philos. 2695. Cf. also Ogle, II. p. 149.

[5] Comp. Said Dierdre, " That man only will I love who hath the three colors that I see here, his cheeks red like the blood, and his body as white as the snow " etc. Leahy, I. p. 98. Cf. also Mabinog. p. 194; J. Grimm, *Altd. Wälder,* I. 9, 10; *Märchen,* No. 53 (and especially the note p. 461);

bination in the picturing of feminine beauty.　Cf. ' A brid briȝt
þai ches, As blod opon snowing,' Tris. 1354 ; ' So faire ȝhe was
& briȝt of mod, Ase snow vpon þe rede blod,' Bev. A. 521.
Closely related to this is the rare combination snow and rose.[6]
Cf. ' Whyte as snow ys hur colour, Hur rud radder þen the
rose flour,' Erl. Tol. 199 (and note) ; Launf. M. 241.

　(g) *As white as the lily and as red as the rose,* is of course
by far the most beloved of all comparisons in picturing the
dazzling loveliness of charming women and fair children.　This
obvious combination is traditional, being found in almost every
literature of the world, and is already in M. E. literature a
stereotyped form of description which is inherited by later
English literature.[7]　As early as Giraldus Cambrensis, snow
and a rosy color play no small part in the description of Eve;

> Lilia puniceo vernant comitata rubore,
> Cum niveo roseus certat in ore color,　Gir. Cam. i. 349.

Cf. further ' Whit so any lili flour, So rose red was hys colour '
(Horn. Child), Horn. 15 ; Athel. 70 ; ' Lylie whyt hue is, hire
rode so rose on rys,' Bödd. W. L. iii. 31 ; Gowth. A. 34 ; Rol.
& Ot. 619 ; Launf. R. 59 ; ' I was radder of rode þene rose in
þe rone, My lere as þe lele,' Awn. Arth. 161 ; Lyd. ii. 5031 ;
iv. 585 ; ii. 3667 ; Horst. C. Misc. 8. 842.

Thurneysen, *Sagen aus Ireland,* p. 14.　For many like quotations from the
German cf. Wackernagel, *op. cit.* p. 155; Schultz, *op. cit.* i. 214.　' White
and red as blood ' is also found in the German, cf. Wackernagel, *op. cit.*
155; and the Virgin Mary is called " ein rôtez helfenbein," cf. Wackernagel,
op. cit. p. 157.

　[6] Very rare . . . found a few times in the Latin and Greek, cf. Ogle i. p.
149.　Cf. Lüdtke to Erl. Tol. 199.　Chaucer gives the only example of
" apple-cheeked " found in M. E. literature (Rom. Rose, 820).　For quotations from the Latin, Greek, and later English cf. Ogle, i. p. 150 f.

　[7] For the Latin, cf. Blümmner, *op. cit.* pp. 60, 160, 185; Old Fr. cf. Loubier, *op. cit.* p. 71; German, cf. Wackernagel, *op. cit.* p. 207; Schultz, *op.
cit.* i. 214.　Comp. Chaucer, C. T., A. 1035; Leahy, i. p. 92; Schick to Lyd's
Temple of Glass, 275; Kaluza to Lib. Des. Intro. civ.　For Spenser's time
cf. Heise, *op. cit.* pp. 35, 119.　Prof. Ogle (*Amer Jour. of Philol.* 34. p.
147) traces the rose-lily conceit from late English back thru the Old Fr.
and Italian to the Classical Latin.　It may be noted that the conceit is
rarely found in the English, French, and Italian sonneteers. p. 148.

Painting. If Nature denied to the women of England the coveted pink-and-white complexion so highly praised by the poets and so in accordance with the taste of the times, they, like the ladies of France, Germany, and Italy, had recourse to all kinds of cosmetics. Strutt (*op. cit.* ii. p. 132) quotes from the *Book of Health* (13th cent.) giving a long recipe for the making of a lotion useful for " cleaning the face, and to give it a beautiful color, either white or red." References to the custom of painting the face are not common in the romances and legends, but wherever it is mentioned, it is in terms of the strongest condemnation. Strutt (*op. cit.* p. 132, ii.), quoting from ms. Harl. 1764, tells of a knight who, in order to prevent his fair daughters from painting their faces, recounts a horrible legend of a fair lady who was punished in hell because she " popped " her face to please the world. The author of Cur. Mun. reproves the belles of his time because they are always studying " Hu to dub and hu to paynt " (28014). Cf. further Sc. Leg. 34. 98; Dest. Tr. 433; Alis. L. 4108; Chaucer, Rom. Rose, 1019. That the paint generally used is white as among the Germans, and not red as among the French and Italians,[8] is suggested by Robert of Brunne's vehement denunciation of the sins of his time, in one passage of which he speaks of those that are so " foule and fade " that they make themselves fairer than God made them " with oblaunchere or ouþer floure, To make hem whytter of coloure," Handlyng Synne, 3217 ff.

Blushes. Inward emotions, such as anger, sympathy, shame, astonishment, and especially the tender emotion of love find outward expression in hot suffusions of the face with blood. Often not the least charming part of a love-scene is the description of the blushes of the fair lady while she is being wooed by her lover. Even in the first love-scene it is said that Eve *Pingitur in vultu pallor ruborque vicissium,* Gir. Cam. i. 353. Cf.

---

[8] Weinhold DF. mentions the custom among English women of painting the face white, cf. p. 224. Wackernagel says (*op. cit.* p. 159) that the German women also used white paint because of their naturally red complexions. For the use of red paint in France and Italy, cf. Weinhold DF. 224; Wackernagel, *op. cit.* p. 159; Buckhardt, *op. cit.* p. 368.

Dest. Tr. 451; Eger & Gr. 1180; Gener. 5173; Gower, iv. 185;
Parton. 11915; Grail. Ap. 129.

Anger. Men in anger are said to become red in the face.
Cf. Gir. Cam. v. 303; Conq. Ire. 88; La3. 1889, 19888; Marh.
fol. 53. a8: Parton. 12064.

Sympathy for her old father makes Cordelia wax " reode on
hire benche, swilche hit were of wine scenche," La3. 3528.

Shame for his weakness causes Sir Gawain to blush pain-
fully, Gaw. & Gr. Kn. 2371, 2503; cf. Gower v. 5988. This
alternation of white and red in the face under emotional excitement is sometimes described as ' change of colour,' ' change
of hue,' or ' out of colour.' Cf. ' Begayn to chaunge her fare
coloure,' Kn. of Cour. 99; Rich. 5938; Ferum. 2925; Boc. i.
269; ' begunne to chaunge her hewe,' Rich. 3445; Sev. Sag.
3902; Oct. S. 95; Boc. iii. 290; Ferum. 2184; Alis. L. 7315,
6871; Sev. Sag. 1902.

Pallor. Pale, faded, discolored faces are never considered
beautiful, probably because pallor is so closely associated with
sorrow, suffering, anger, fear, death, and especially with dis-
appointed love.[9]   Pallor may result from,

(a) *Wounds received in battle.* Cf. ' al discolourid . . . for
is blod was gon away,' Ferum. 1079, 290; ' pale of hewe,'
Ferum. 294, 332, 772, 780, 922. The verb *fealwen* (cf. further Willms, *op. cit.* p. 38) is sometimes used to describe faces
becoming pale in battle. Cf. ' falewede nebbes,' La3. 4163,
23214, 26812, 30414, 30987; Mort. Arth. 3954; Rich. 4807.
The verb *blakien* [10] and the adjective *blāc,* meaning to turn pale
and pale, are found many times. Cf. ' þat hæfde bledde, ah
he ne blakede no, for he wes cniht wel idon,' La3. 7524; ' What
for buffetis and blode here blees wex blake,' Awn. Arth. 658;
cf. Guy. B. 4654, 4286; Dest. Tr. 9132.

(b), *Fear.* Cf. ' hire bleo bigont to blakien,' Marh. fol. 44,

----

[9] For further discussion of pallor cf. Willms, *op. cit.* pp. 36-40, 53-63;
Mead, *P. M. L. A.* 14. p. 177. Comp. also Blümmner, *op. cit.* pp. 83, 85,
86, 88, 129.

[10] Madden in the gloss to La3. renders the verb ' to become black,' but
cf. Stratt-Brad. and Mead, *P. M. L. A.* 14. p. 177.

a15; Pier. Lang. 4505, 6039; Boc. I. 462; i. 241, 272; Trev.
VII. 195; Horst. C. Misc. 4. 756; Havel. 2165; Alis C. 5302;
Grail. 15. 638; 9. 18; 'To blake þo bigan her brewes,' Cur.
Mun. 14746, 17430; Avow. Arth. xv; Perc. Gal. 688 (and
Note), 1056; Torr. 236.

(c), *Anger*. Cf. 'For angre sche wax al pal,' Ferum. 2015;
Gener. 3349; Dest. Tr. 11015, Pist. Sus. 303; Laȝ. 3069. If
the martyrs do not die easily under the first few tortures, it is
right and customary for the wicked judges to wax pale with
anger. Cf. Horst. C. 22. 325; Boc. 12. 427; 7. 126; 3. 555.

(d), *Unrequited or unsatisfied love*. If the course of true
love does not run smoothly, both the knight and his lady are
conventionally bound to appear before their friends pale and
disconsolate. When she falls in love, "Bresaid, the bright,
blackonet of hew," Dest. Tr. 8038. Cf. *ibid.* 493; Kn. of Cour
69; Squyr. 711; Gener. 750; Erl. Tol. 496 (knight), 643;
Gener. 764, 4702; Iw. & Gaw. 913; Parton. 6654, 7401, 6661,
7289.

(e), *Sorrow and grief*. For sorrow cf. Cur. Mun. 24003;
Gol. & Gaw. 1133; Bon. Flor. 587; Dest. Tr. 9134; 'pale as
any stone,' Squyr. 711; 'chekis . . . þat falow were & fad,'
Sc. Leg. 41. 47; Gener. 6759, 1296; Guy. B. 284; R. Brunn.
2510; Max. 30; Beryn. 951; Parton. 8656; Gregor. V. 1068.

(f), *Suffering, sickness, and death*. Cf. 'falow & fade,' Sc.
Leg. 32. 396; 'wan in face,' Cur. Mun. 4757; 'pale as eny
leed,' Horst. B. Misc. 5. 521; Sc. Leg. 34. 317; Horst. C. Misc.
19. 88; Horst. D. 59. 134; 'þi face es wann sua rose vnred'
(Christ), Cur. Mun. 24471; Trev. III. 371. The livid, ghastly
pallor of dying or dead bodies is described by the adjectives
pale, wan, blue, and black. Cf. 'his neb bigon to blakien,'
Laȝ. 19799; 'Wex pale of his payne,' Dest. Tr. 13919; 'waxed
bloo as any ledde,' Guy. B. 4667; Thos. Ercel. 135; Max. 212;
'þi neb al blo,' Guy. A. 4884, 506; 'lady blew and wan,' Am.
& Am. 2458; Bödd. G. L. xi. 24; Max. 212; 'His body wexe
als bla als lede,' Horst. C. Misc. 22. 525; 'And alle the blee of
his body wos blakke as þe moldes,' Horst. C. Misc. 343; 'blak
and blo' (Christ), Bödd. G. L. VIII. 17. Ghosts have a par-

7

ticularly ghastly appearance. Cf. 'Sancte Nicholas to þame
aperyt bla & bludy,' Sc. Leg. 26. 929, 961; 'body . . . blake
to þe bone,' Awn. Arth. 105; 'body es blakonede so bare,' Awn.
Arth. 203, 212; 'mi soule is won so is þe led,' Bödd. G. L. x.
13; Trev. viii. 46. Bodies that are beaten and bruised are said
to be black or blue. Cf. 'And made his body al blo' Isum.
298; Horst. B. p. 205, 1. 76; *ibid.* C. 248. 281; Feurm. 2908;
Awn. Arth. 658 (cf. further Willms, *op. cit.* p. 15, 63).

(g), *Hunger and old age.* Cf. 'feynt & pal for hungre &
for þerst,' Ferum. 2830, 2822; Havel. 470; 'Thei weren pale
and fade hewed' (age), Gower, i. 2043.

Certain combinations and comparisons are used to emphasize
the pallor of persons described. Cf. 'Pale and wan,' Iw. &
Gaw. 913; Guy. B. 284, 4654, 4286; Gregor. A. 731; V. 1006;
R. 404; C. 834; Horst. C. Misc. 4. 756; Gener. 750, 1296,
4702, 6759; Ipom. 196 (and note); Beryn. 1819, 3524; 'his
visage waxed pan and wale,' Eger. & Gr. 1082; (cf. further
Schick to Lyd's. Temple of Glass and Mead, *op. cit.* p. 326);
'pale and grene,' Bev. M. 3875; Gregor. A. 751 'ȝelew and
grene,' Bev. E. 3883; Eger. & Gr. 69; ' pale and bleche,' Gower,
v. 2477; 'grene and bleike,' Havel. 470; 'wone and wonder
grene,' Gregor. C. 853; 'falu . . . & won,' Max. 228; 'so pal
so clay,' Ferum. 81; 'lyke þe pale asshe,' Parton. 7401, 6654;
' So muchel y þenke upon þe þat al y woxe grene,' Bödd. W. L.
xii. 16; G. L. vi. 11; Beryn. 2132 (cf. Willms, *op. cit.* p. 54).

An oft recurring circumlocution or paraphrase, referring to
the appearance of the skin and complexion in general, is the
expression 'hide and hew.' Cf. 'Scho was ful faire of hide
and hew,' Horst. C. 10.3; 18. 5; 27. 60, 373; Eger. & Gr. 263;
Erl. Tol. 188; 'Ladye louesome of hew and hyde,' Eger. & Gr.
851; Parton. Frag. 12. Noble knights are also " faire of hewe
and hide," Rol. & Ot. 65, 1171, 1230; Triam. C. 468; Rich.
675; Dest. Tr. 3908. Sometimes sorrow causes a change of
' hide and hew ' i. e. pallor. Cf. Tars. 368 Le Mort. Arth. 3757
and note; Squyr. 387; Iw. & Gaw. 885. For ugly people with
loathly ' hide and hew ' cf. Ferum. 4465; Rich. 675; Rol. & Ot.
1460.

§ 16. HEAD.

Of the head in general the poet seldom takes occasion to speak; he loves rather to describe the individual parts of it. If not too large, however, a capacious head is greatly admired. Of the skull of King Arthur it is said, *Os etiam capitis tanquam ad prodigium vel ostentum capax erat et grossum* (Gir. Cam. viii. 129), and Henry II. is described with *amplo capite et rotundo* (Gir. Cam. v. 303; cf. Conq. Ire. 88; Trev. viii. 22). A very large, thick head is considered ugly. Geoffrey, Archb. of York, is *capite grosso* (Gir. Cam. iv. 420), Alagolafre the giant has a " grete harde hede " (Sow. Bab. 2902), and the head of other giants are compared to those of horses, cattle, leopards, and boars. Cf. ' Hyt was so oryble & so greet, More þan any Horse heed,' Arth. 393; ' With bores hede, blake and donne,' Sow. Bab. 346; ' And hede like an libarde,' Sow. Bab. 2192, 2198; ' His hevyd . . . was als grete Als of a rowncy or a nete,' Iw. & Gaw. 251.

§ 17. NECK.

Fair maidens " swete of Swyre " appear in Seg. Mely. 36; Bon. Flor. 440; Bödd. W. L. x. 27. Sir Gawain has a " fayre hals " (Gaw. & Gr. Kn. 1388), and when he goes to receive the borrowed stroke, he leans the neck a little " & schewed þat schyre al bare," *ibid.* 2255.

In shape the neck of a beautiful woman should be small, round, so long as to be compared to that of a swan, and so plump that no bone may be seen.[1] Of Eve we are told,

Colli forma teres et longa desenter et ampla,
Sustinet hoc tanquam fida columna caput, Gir. Cam. i. 350.

---

[1] Comp. Chaucer, Duchess, 940;

But swich a fairnesse of a nekke
Had that swete, that boon nor brekke
Nas ther non sene, that mis-sat.

Cf. further, 'Swannes swyre swyþe wel y-sette, A sponne len-
gore þen y mette,' Bödd. W. L. v. 45; 'Her swere long &
small,' Lib. Des. 946; 'He seth hire neck round and clene,
Thereinne mai no bon be sene,' Gower, vi. 777. The white
neck is an especial characteristic of feminine loveliness,[2] and is
occasionally ascribed to handsome men. Cf. 'yee leudis wit
your quite hals,' Cur. Mun. 29010 ' white swere,' Tars. 16; Awn.
Arth. L. 713; Gower, iv. 859; viii. 116; Guy. C. 71; 'nekke
feyr & whyt,' Boc. 9. 1024; 'hir bright swire,' Dest. Tr. 9036;
' hur necke full scheene,' Alis. A. 185; 'Hys neck was feyre,
whyte and longe' (fair knight), Alis. L. 2000. Conventional
comparisons are used to express the brilliancy of the white neck.
Cf. 'hire faire hals . . . *mylk-quhyt*,' Sc. Leg. 50. 1172;
'mylky nekkes beeþ i-wasche wiþ gold,' Trev. i. 267 (This characteristic of the Gallic race is mentioned also by Blümmner, *op.
cit.* p. 40), '*Here swyre was whyt as ony swan*,' Horst. C. Misc.
4. 752; Bödd. W. L. ii. 28; 'hir bryȝt þrote . . . *Schon
schyrer þen snawe*,[3] þat schedes on hilleȝ,' Gaw. & Gr. Kn. 955.
Helen is shown to be the very flower of beauty,

> With a necke for þe nonest of naturs deuyse,
> Glissonand as the glemes þat glenttes of þe snaw;
> Nawþer fulsom, ne fat, but fetis & round,
> ffull metely made of a meane lenght,   Dest. Tr. 3066.

> Hit was whyt, smothe, streght and flat,
> Withouten hole; and canel-boon,
> As by seming, had she noon.

Cf. also Rom. Rose. 551. So in the O. Fr. cf. Loubier, *op. cit.* p. 96; Voigt,
op. cit. p. 60; in the German, cf. Schultz, *op. cit.* i. 216; comp. Sec. Sec.
227, 116, "A longe neke and not ouer grete tokenyth corageous like a
lyon "; cf. Philos. p. 85.

[2] So in other languages, cf. Blümmner, *op. cit.* p. 22; Loubier, *op. cit.* p.
96; Schultz, *op. cit.* i. p. 216; Weinhold, DF. i. 227. Comp. Mead, A. p. 179.

[3] Comp. Chaucer, Rom. Rose, 557, 'Hir throte also white of hewe As
snowe on braunche snowed newe'; Troil. i. 1250; Willms, *op. cit.* p. 21.
Cf. also Ott, *op. cit.* p. 7; Loubier, *op. cit.* p. 96; Voigt, *op. cit.* p. 60;
Weinhold AL. p. 31; and Blümmner, *op. cit.* p. 35 for like comparison in
the Fr. Germ. and Latin. Blümmner also presents *ivory* as an object of
comparison, cf. *op. cit.* p. 40, with which we may compare Chaucer's Duchesse, 'Hir throte . . . Semed a round tour of yvoire,' Bk. of Duch. 945.
Cf. in addition the Frere of Chaucer, 'His nekke whyt was as the flour-
de-lys,' C. T., A. 239.

The skin of the neck should be of such transparent whiteness that the red wine which the lovely one drinks may be seen thru it.[4] Adler will love only that maiden who is as soft as silk, as white as any milk, ' *the royall rich wine runes downe her brest bone,*' Adler, 7, 12. (For a ' *lyly-whyte* ' neck, cf. Parton. 5160).

The short, thick neck is exceedingly ugly. Three times Giraldus Cambrensis describes his wicked or ugly men with *collo contracto* (Gir. Cam. v. 272, 354; IV. 420; cf. Conq. Ire. 54), and even king Henry II. is *collo ab humeris aliquantulum demisso,* Gir. Cam. v. 303 (cf. Conq. Ire. 88). Cf. ' Schorte y-swerred,' Alis. L. 6264; ' neke as an ape ' (giant), Ipom. A. 6162; ' Bullenekkyde was þat bierne ' (cannibal), Mort. Arth. 1094; ' He ne had noither nekke ne throte, His heued was in his body y-chote,' Alis. L. 5952. The loathly Dame Ragnell has a short neck in Gower (I. 1687), and indeed it is further said of her that, " Nek forsothe on her was none iseen,' Wed. Gaw. 556.

A black rough neck is also considered ugly. The Devil is said to have a " ruhe necke " (Marh. fol. 46, b16), and when Horn disguises himself, he " al bicolmede his swere, He makede him vn-bicomelich," Horn. 1143.

§ 17. FORM, FIGURE, STATURE.

Women. The figures of women should be fair (*avenand, hende*), seemly, well-formed and perfectly well-proportioned, of a delicate gracefulness (*small*) and of aristocratic elegance (*gent, gentil*), tall and stately. Cf. ' feyre bodye,' Bon. Flor. 1515; Gaw. & Gr. Kn. 943; ' Of body sche was ful auenaunt,' R. Brunn. 7599, 10421; ' Semely of a Sise,' Dest. Tr. 3993; Lyd. II. 4999; ' joure semely doujter, how fair, how fetis she is, how freli schapen,' Wm. Palern. 126, 1447; Erl. Tol. 346; ' sche is made withouten lak,' Oph. 422; ' Florence worthlyly

---

[4] The same conceit is found in the German, cf. Weinhold DF. I. 227; Schultz, *op. cit.* I. p. 216.

wroght,' Bon. Flor. 1091, 107, 1846; 'hir bodye well sette and
shaply,' Guy. C. 73; 'of shape both faire and trim,' Horst, C.
Misc. 24. 13; 'of body *fair and gent*,' Alis. L. 5006; Ferum,
2473; Emar. 191, 403; Bev. O. 3602; Iw. & Gaw. 1423; R.
Brunn. 3166; Arth. & Merl. 478; Am. & Am. 1766; Rol. & Ot.
1144; Guy. B. 2146; Arth. 358; Thos. Ercel. 255; Torr. F.
205, 1837.

Gent. Noble birth and good breeding show in every line of a
woman's form. As the poet says; " Gentelri is plaunt, as y ʒow
telle, In wiman is springeþ in ich a liʒþ," Lob. Frau. 56. This
elegance of figure is expressed innumerable times by the word
gent, or *gentil* which, like fair, appears upon every possible
occasion. Cf. 'lady gent,' Emar. 932, etc.; 'Gentyl of body,'
R. Brunn. 5574; 'Gentil, iolyf so þe joy,' Bödd. W. L. x. 41;
' The gentileste jowelle a-juggede with lordes,' Mort. Arth. 862;
' Hure body iantil and pure fetys, & semblych of stature,'
Ferum. 5883; 'Hyr body was gentyll withouten lacke,' Bev. O.
401. Gent occurs often in compounds. Cf. ' Dame, *gent and
fre*,' Sev. Sag. 625, 2587, 2749; Sow. Bab. 1628; ' *gentil &
auenaunt*,' R. Brunn. 15680; ' *gent & precious*,' Arth. & Merl.
4474; ' *Gentyl and amyable*,' Kn. of Cour. 6; ' *gent and rody*,'
Arth. & Merl. 654.

Small in the sense of slender, graceful (*gracilis*) occurs alone
and in various combinations. Cf. ' maydens faire smal,' Ferum.
1737; Horst. B. Misc. 6. 141; Rol. & Ot. 427; Bon. Flor. 52;
Amad. 585; Torr. 245; Sc. Leg. 1. 50, 277. The combination
gent and small is especially beloved. Cf. ' To se her bak and
side, How gent sche was and small,' Lib. Des. 928; ' douʒtir
smal & gent,' Cur. Mun. 13138; Iw. & Gaw. 899; Gowth. A.
690; Bon. Flor. 393, 479; Sev. Sag. 2647; 'gentylle and
smalle,' Emar. 391; Erl. Tol. 701; (comp. Chaucer, C. T., A.
3233, 'As any wesele hir body gent and small); ' *Long, small
and well farynge*,' Guy. A. 57; ' bodies long and smal,' Gower,
iv. 1320; Lyd. ii. 1703; ' Longe of hir schap . . . angelik of
figure,' Lyd. ii. 4982; Dest. Tr. 3984; (comp. Chaucer, C. T.,
B. 3263, ' Long as mast and upright as a bolt'). After the
smiths' wife has been made over, it is said that there is none in

Egypt her peer, " So fayre and so tall " (Sc. Leg. 28, 23), another beautiful lady has a " bodi round " (Gower, vi. 786), and an ideal wife is a " leath maiden . . . as softe as any silke " (Adler, 8, 15). The Amazons of course " were strong of hor stature " (Dest. Tr. 10812), and Hecuba " Was shewyng in shap of a shene brede, Massily made as a man lyke " (Dest. Tr. 3974).

As to the exact stature of women desired it is hard to say anything definite. But the original pattern of all womanhood, Eve, is reported to have been taller than medium, and lower than the very tall (Gir. Cam. i. 350). Cressid is neither " To hi3e nor lowe, but mene of stature " (Lyd. ii. 4740), and Helen is described,

> Hir corse was comly & of clene shap,
> Euyn metely made of a medill deuyse
> As nobly to þe nethur-most as nature cold shape,
>
> Dest. Tr. 3082.[1]

As for ugly figures, those that are short and thick (Gaw. & Gr. Kn. 966), or large without slenderness and grace (Gower, i. 1689; comp. Chaucer, C. T., A. 3973) are looked upon with disgust.

Men. Men should be well-formed, large of body, massively built, broad, thick, strong in battle, with aristocratic grace and ease of movement. Cf. ' faire of schap,' R. Brunn. 7312, 7298, 14403 ; ' Of faire stature wyþouten lak,' R. Brunn. 7291 ; ' body . . . of fare stature,' Sc. Leg. 7. 765 ; 'how fair, how fetys it was & freliche schapen,' Wm. Paler. 225, 393 ; ' wiþouten last al his licame,' Cur. Mun. 22324 ; ' their comli shape,' Horst. C. 24. 927 ; Gener. 1907 ; ' of pure shap, Semely for sothe, & of Syse faire,' Dest. Tr. 3814 ; ' Stronge of his stature,' Dest. Tr. 3794 ; ' wele made in alle wyse,' Per. Gal. 1258 ; Ferum. 1847 ; Barb. i. 387 ; ' A bettir compact was ther noon alyue, Nor pro-

---

[1] The persons of beautiful women are supposed to be made more attractive by the use of perfume. Cf. Sc. Leg. 34. 33 ; Cur. Mun. 9356. Wright tells us that " The art of perfuming is said to have been practised throughout the East from a very remote date, and it seems to have been brought thence into Western Europe," *op. cit.* p. 242. The favorite perfume of feudal ladies was saffron.

porcyownyd of fetures nor stature,' Horst. C. Misc. 20a.-86;
' Ful wel compact,' Lyd. ii. 4609; 4623, 4951; ' Merion . . .
was massely shapen, A faire man of fourme, & a fre knyght,'
Dest. Tr. 3963; ' Troilus þe tru was full tore mekull, Full
massely made, & of mayn strenght,' Dest. Tr. 3922, 3885, 6173;
Gol. & Gaw. 614; ' biostous fourme and ded strong,' Horst.
D. 45. 672; ' Off his persone and off his stature, was noon so
likly that tyme,' Horst. C. Misc. 20c. 302; ' Body stalwart and
strang,' Gol. & Gaw. 89; R. Brunn. 5896; Torr. 2396; ' In al
þe londe was þer non hold So faire of boon ne blode,' Am. Am.
59; Havel. 344; ' He was burely,[2] of body and thereto riȝt brade,'
Perc. Gal. 269; ' He was borlich and bigge, Pist. Sus. 226; Lyd.
ii. 4639; ' Agamemnon þe gay was of a gode mykull . . . He
was store man of strenght,' Dest. Tr. 3741; ' Nis in al þis kine-
lond, cniht swa muchel ne swa strong,' Laȝ. 13896; ' He was
mekyll of boon and lyth,' Triam. C. 467; ' Feyre and grete and
moche he was,' Guy. B. 4281.

Knights are often described as being large, huge, or big. Cf.
' *Large he was of leme and lyth,*' Ipom. A. 40, 361; Dest. Tr.
3818; Parton. 9204, 9396; Orph. 27; Grail. 13. 647; ' large of
blood and bone,' Eger. & Gr. 29, 1151, 1225; ' *þat vnsely hoge
man,*' Arth. & Merl. 6284; Gaw. & Gr. Kn. 844; ' Of huge
makyng & also of gret strengþe, Wel answeryng his brede to his
lengþe,' Lyd. ii. 4563; Dest. Tr. 3768; ' *Begge he wex of bonne
& blode,*' Ipom. A. 52, 762, 2593, 7670; Torr. 1714; Gol. &
Gaw. 6; Gener. 2074; Havel. 1174; Gaw. & Gr. Kn. 554;
Dest. Tr. 4116, 5485; Pist. Sus. 226; ' body bigger þen þe best
fowre þat ar in Arþureȝ hous,' Gaw. & Gr. Kn. 2100; ' Half
elayn in erde I hope þat he were,' Gaw. & Gr. Kn. 140. (For
great warriors compared to giants, cf. Skeat's Chaucer. Vol. v.
p. 191; Wülfing, *Anglia,* 28. p. 45).

Historical characters. The chronicles, especially the Latin,
abound in appreciative descriptions of large, strong, and well-

---

[2] For the original meaning of burly, " suitable for a lady's bower," cf.
W. W. Skeat, *Acad.* Vol. 45. 1142, p. 250. In the quotations here given,
however, the word seems to have taken on the meaning which it has today.

formed historical characters. Cf. *corpore peramplo* (Dermot), Gir. Cam. v. 238; *corpore pervalido* (Wm. Rufus), Gir. Cam. v. 344 (cf. Conq. Ire. 118); *corpore quadrato,* Wm. Malms. 5049 (cf. R. Glouc. 8571, ' þikke mon he was ynou round . . . wel iboned & strong '); *corpore tamen pro quantitatis captu pervalido* (Meiler), Gir. Cam. v. 324 (cf. Conq. Ire. 99); *corpore procero* (Rich. of Striguil), Gir. Cam. v. 272 (Cf. Conq. Ire. 54); *amplo corpore et integro,* Gir. Cam. v. 272 (cf. Conq. Ire. 54); *corpore . . . valde venustos,* Hen. Hunt. 76; *pulcherrimis et proceris corporibus* (Irish), Gir. Cam. v. 150; *formae nitore praeclarus* (Giraldus), Gir. Cam. iv. 104; *pro corporis captu habitudine bona, ad tenuitatem tamen quam ad corpulentiam magis accommoda* (Baldwin), Gir. Cam. vi. 148; v. 323 (cf. Conq. Ire. 98); 'Vair mon & þikke inou,' R. Glouc. 8841 (Hen. I.); 'Suiþ þikke mon he was & of grete strengþe,' (Wm. Conqueror), R. Glouc. 7730.[3]

That giants are of enormous size goes almost without saying; but their hugeness does not necessarily carry with it the idea of ugliness. While the bigness and strength of the hero is described in order to excite admiration, the loathly bulk of the giant enemy, whom he always overcomes, is given to excite wonder. Giants are sometimes compared to oxen, horses, and oaks in size and strength. Cf. ' Hys breste was brode, his body grete, He was thykker than a nete,' Guy. C. 7761; Guy. G. 7581; 'He was so large and so grett, That no hors hym bere myght,' Guy. B. 10220; Gener. 2155; Torr. 1268; Grail. 37. 103; ' Greet as an ok,' Oct. S. 922; R. Glouc. 4240.

Stature. As the valiant hero of a stirring romance, a man of low or medium stature is of rare occurrence. I have found only three of mean height who are described with approval, and two of these are Greek heroes. Cf. ' Þou art euenliche long' (Horn), Horn. 99, 969; 'Machoon . . . was of a mene sta-

---

[3] That a feminine delicacy of person was not appreciated is suggested by the fact that Wm. Malms. rails against the hateful customs in vogue in the reign of Wm. Rufus when *molitie corporis cetare cum foeminis . . . adolescentium specimen erat.* Wm. Malms. p. 498.

ture, Noght to long ne to litle,' Dest. Tr. 3845; Lyd. ii. 4670;
'But Menelay of stature was but mene, Proporcioned atwixe
schort and longe,' Lyd. ii. 4542; Dest. Tr. 3749. The Christ,
however, an ideal man of the religious world, is said to have
been of mean stature; " Of heiȝte he was a metely mon . . .
Nouþer to grete ny to smal," Cur. Mun. 18827, and His faithful follower, St. Bartholomew, is *statura aequalis quae nec longa
possit, nec brevis adverti,* Gir. Cam. ii. 68 (comp. corresponding passages, Horst. C. 24. 92; Sc. Leg. 9. 53; Horst. D. 55.
62).

On the contrary, most of the kings and other personages
found in the chronicles are of but mean stature.   Cf. *statura
minimos supergrediens, a maximis vincebatur* (Hen. I.), Wm.
Malms. 642 (cf. R. Glouc. 8840); *Justae fuit staturæ* (Wm.
Conqueror), Wm. Malms. 478 (cf. R. Glouc. 7731); *non mag-
nae staturae* (Wm. Rufus), Wm. Malms. 504; *ibid.* 213; *Staturae vir erat inter mediocres* (Henry II.), Gir. Cam. v. 303;
Trev. viii. 24; *Erat . . . staturae . . . paulo plus quas mediocris* (Reimund f. Gerald), Gir. Cam. v. 323 (cf. Conq. Ire.
98); *statura paulo mediocritem excedente* (Robt. f. Stephen),
Gir. Cam. v. 272 (cf. Conq. Ire. 54); *tam staturae quam fac-
turae inter parum mediocribus majores satis idonae* (Wm. f.
Audeline), Gir. Cam. v. 337 (cf. Conq. Ire. 112); *staturae
paulo mediocri plus pusillae* (Meiler), Gir. Cam. v. 324 (cf.
Conq. Ire. 99); Gir. Cam. v. 199, 297 (cf. Conq. Ire. 76);
vir . . . inclytus, cujus statura mediocriter eminens (Frederick I.), Gir. Cam. viii. 279; *statura modica* (Baldwin), Gir.
Cam. vi. 148; *Abbas Samson mediocris erat staturae,* Joc. Brak.
29; 'He wes of mesurabil stature' (Thos. Randolph), Barb. x.
280.   I have found only five historical characters whose exceptional height is considered worth mentioning.   Cf. *Eram . . .
statura procerus* (Giraldus Cam.), Gir. Cam. iv. 104; *staturae
grandis* (Dermot and John of Courci), Gir. Cam. v. 344, 238
(cf. Conq. Ire. 118); *statura pergrandem* (Bishop Walkerus),
Higd.-Trev. vii. 266; *vir longae staturae paululum incurvus*
(Paulinus), Hen. Hunt. 87.

This general mediocrity of stature, which seems to be a common and natural characteristic of the race, is probably responsible for the excessive homage and worship paid to the men of exceptional height and elegance of person. The ideal hero of the romances is always tall and stately, looking down upon those about him, and exciting admiration by his strength and prowess. He is most often described as being 'great and long.' Cf. 'cniht he wes swiðe strong, Kene and custi, muchel and long,' Laȝ. 63666; Horn. Ch. 290, 295; 'He was long man and heye,' Isum. 36; 'body long,' Alis. L. 2002, 7351; 'a moche man and a longe,' Triam. C. 615; 'long man and hende,' Thos. Ercel. L. 291; Ferum. 1352; Parton, 2525; 'wandirly brade & lange,' Horst. C. Misc. 22, 27; 'mekill of brede and lenth,' Horst. C. 26. 103; Horst. D. 40. 81; Max. 253; Guy. C. 7910, 8051; Guy. B. 7725, 4291, 10154, 10827, 2821; Oct. S. 1011; 'Long man & large,' Dest. Tr. 3947, 3864, 3805, 3756, 3760; Troy H. 1082; Lyd. II. 2757. 'lengest of stature,' Lyd. II. 4623, 4609; 'Of largenes & lenght no lesse þen a giaund,' Dest. Tr. 5503, 6173; Lyd. II. 4792; 'An huge man of lengþe,' Ferum. 5489. Havelok, the ideal English knight,[4] is so "þicke in þe brest, of bodi long' that he stands above other warriors head and shoulders (Havel. 1699), or towers above them like a mast (Havel. 986, 2242).

The clean-cut, slim, graceful, manly figure of high-bred elegance is also highly appreciated. Cf. 'Priam þe prise kyng was of pure shap, A large man & a longe, liuely & small,' Dest. Tr. 3864 (cf. Guido, *longe fuisse stature, gracilem et decorum,* sig. e₂ recto 2); Anthenor 'Was sclendre & longe,' Lyd. II. 4929 (cf. Guido, *fuit longus et gracilis,* sig. e₂ verso 2); Palamedes was 'of body longe and lene,' Lyd. II. 4654 (cf. Guido, *fuit longus et gracilis,* sig. e₂ recto 2); Dest. Tr. 3830, 3855, 3864, 3959; Sev. Sav. 54.

The adjectives 'high' and 'tall' are sometimes used to de-

---

[4] Comp. here a fine description of King Arthur taken from MS. Ashmole 802, fol. 56, and of Sir Gawain from the same MS. quoted by Halliwell, *Thornton Romances,* pp. 257, 263.

scribe men of great stature. Cf. 'A muchel mon of stature
heȝe,' Cur. Mun. 23321; Trist. 1222; Erl. Tol. 1000; Isum. 16;
'bothe large and heghe,' Isum. C. 244, 13; Lyd. ii. 4532, 4864,
4781, 4577, 4554; Dest. Tr. 6153, 6615; 'Of stature had he
sene none more,' Horst. C. 6234; Dest. Tr. 12268; Lyd. ii. 4951.
It is said that King Saul " Was heȝer þen any man, Bi þe schuldres founden þan " (Cur. Mun. 7331), of Golagrus that " Thair
wes na hathill sa heich, be half ane fute hicht " (Gol. & Gaw.
900), and the famous Green Knight is "On þe most on þe
molde on mesure hyghe " (Gaw. & Gr. Kn. 136).

We find also something of a definite character concerning the
stature of gigantic heroes of romance and legend. The information, however, seems to depend entirely in its variableness
upon the mood the poet happens to be in, upon his enthusiasm,
and upon the degree of admiration he desires to awaken for his
noble knight. For instance, in Trev. (vi. 253) we are informed
that Charles the Great " was eyte foot of lenhþe," but the ro-
mancer will not have it so, rather " Tventi fete he was o lengþe,
& al so of gret strengþe " (Rol. & Varn. 431). Reports vary
still more as to the height of the wonderfully broad and 'long '
St. Christopher. In one place we are told that " twelf cubitis
he had of hicht " (Sc. Leg. 19. 27); in another " Foure-and-
twenti fet he was long " (Horst. D. 40. 3); and an evidently
very imaginative legend writer gives him thirty feet, " Twentty
cubettes he was of heghte " (Horst. C. Misc. 22. 27). Alexander was " Thre cubettis fra þe croune doun " (Alis. C. 3987),
and " þe person of ser Porrus past him þat hiȝt twyse " (*ibid.*
3988). The famous Butcher of Paris as " þe frensch seyð
. . . was of heȝt Ten foot of length " (Oct. S. 407). The
height of the leaders of the Saracen hosts against whom Arthur
and his men have to fight varies from fourteen to seventeen feet.
How great is Arthur to overcome such valiant men! Cf. 'Ai-
þer of hem was xiiii fot long,' Arth. & Merl. 6050, 5997, 6181,
8481, 4885; 'Lengþe he hadde o fet fiftene,' Arth. & Merl.
8846, 5968 Ferum. 546; 'Sexten fet o lengþe he was,' Arth. &
Merl. 7748; 'He was seuenten fet long,' Arth. & Merl. 8975.

Giants. That giants are described as being long and high is not surprising. Cf. 'Greet he was & also heȝe, he semed sathanas vnsleȝe,' Cur. Mun. 7445, 7451; 'a geaunt gret & longe,' R. Brunn. 14807; 'the gyant heygh,' Torr. 100; 'The geaunte was bath large and lang,' Iw. & Gaw. 2385; 'This geaunte hade a body longe . . . Therto he was devely stronge,' Sow. Bab. 2191, 353; Guy. C. 8051; Guy. B. 7593; Guy. C. 10319; Guy. B. 7955. Comparative measurements are sometimes given. Cf. 'He ys two fote and more Hyer then any that was þore,' Guy. B. 7558; 'þe lengþe of his body passed the heiȝte of þe walles,' Trev. I. 223.

As to exact and definite height, the giant race seems to vary from ten to forty feet—according to the imaginative quality of the author's mind. The grisly Bishop Longis "hadde in leynthe ten grete feet" (Alis. L. 6817); the terrible Alagolafre was a "Sarsyn of wonder gret Strengþe, XV fet . . . in lengþe" (Ferum. 4329 f.; cf. Lib. Des. 688); of whose children we are told that at four months old they were seven feet and three inches tall (Ferum. 4659); the giant, Gogmagog, was "Twelue cubyte . . . in lengþe" (R. Brun. 1830), or according to R. Glous, "Gogmagog was a geant swiȝe gret & strong, Vor aboute twenti vet me seiþ he was long," R. Glouc. 508 ff. Another loathly son of the Devil "was of lengthe twenty feet, And two elle yn brede" (Oct. S. 925), or according to another account, he "was XX fote and two Betwyx hys hedd and hys too " (Oct. N. 826); while a third, whom Sir Torrent overcomes, measures "XXIII fotte Ther he lay on the þente" (Torr. 678). We are delighted to learn that the cannibal monster in Mort. Arth. (1103) "ffro þe face to þe fote, was fyfe fadome lange," and that the wonderfully strong giant in Bev. A. (1859) was " Rome þretti fote long." (Cf. also *ibid.,* 2508). Surely the Saracen, Vernagu, was the very pink and flower of the giant kind, for " He hadde tventi men strengþe, fourti fet of lengþe þilke panim hede," Rol. & Vern. 473.

Very ugly is the deformed or crooked [5] body, and despicable

---

[5] Persons with deformed bodies are not to be trusted, cf. Philos, 2542;

is a short, thick-set, insignificant stature. Cf. *Si staturam quae-ris exiguus ... corpore piloso pariter et nervoso ... si facturam, deformis,* Gir. Cam. v. 354; *Erat itaque statura exigua despec-taque, et clune claudus utroque,* Gir. Cam. IV. 420; ' His lire and his lyghame lamede fulle sore,' Mort. Arth. 3282; ' crom-pylde and crokyd,' Bon. Flor. 1971. Dwarfs in general are not beautiful because of their deformities and low stature.[6] It is said of one in particular that " 4 foote was they lenght of him, his visage was both gret & grim," Degree P. 645.

In the chronicles, however, if a man is strong and powerful, full of prowess, with a great heart and a brave spirit, his na-tural shortness of stature need count nothing against him. Bishop Rimigius *Erat ... statura parvus, sed corde magnus* (Hen. Hunt. 212), and Balso, a Norman, was a man *exigui corporis sed immanis fortitudinis,* because of which he is said to have gained the nickname, ' the short' (Wm. Malms, 230). Robert Courthose had no defect save that he was not tall, being " þikke and Quarre " enough, but because of his shortness he was dubbed Shorthose (cf. R. Glouc. 8526), and the prowess of Edgar was not to be despised because *staturae fuerit et cor-pulentiae perexilis* (Wm. Malms. 251. Cf. Trev. VI. 467; R. Glouc. 5785). The good knight Robt. of Normandy was a " litel man of body " (Trev. IV. 449; cf. Wm. Malms. 607); so was the ' orped' man, Sabinus (Trev. IV. 499), and even Aeneas was " of body litill,' Dest. Tr. 3936 (Cf. Alis. L. 5499).

Fat. If the slender, well-formed figure is so highly appre-ciated, on the contrary the body fleshy and fat is considered ugly. Cf. ' Greese growene as a galte,' Mort. Arth. 111; ' Poli-darius was pluccid as a porke fat, ffull grete in the grippe, all

Sec. Sec. pp. 114, 232; cf. Horst. D. 66. 209; Mort. Arth. 3282. Comp. Chaucer's Miller, ' He was short-scholdered, broad, a thikke knarre,' C. T., A. 549; cf. Trev. I. p. 53. Men who have a preponderance of the element fire are " smal and red," Horst. D. 45. 686.

[6] The strange blue people of Albanyen are described, " Of foure feet hy habbeth the lengthe " (Alis. L. 5272); the Durwes are " Thikke and schort and gud sette, Ac non so hygh . . . So the leynthe of on elne " (Alis. L. 6267); while certain pigmies are to be found in India, " men of a cubite longe," Trev. I. 81.

of grese hoge, So bolnet was his body; þat burthen hade ynoghe
The fete of þat freke to ferke hym aboute,' Dest. Tr. 3837 (cf.
Lyd. II. 4572, 4645, 4663, 4768). Gower finds that the man
of fat body is slow in spiritual labors (v. 1947), and that it
is hard for him to keep his chastity (I. 474). Among historical
characters who stand out as men of extraordinary corpulency
are Wm. the Conqueror (Wm. Malms. 458; Trev. VII. 314),
Henry II (Gir. Cam. v. 303; Conq. Ire. 88), Henry I. (Wm.
Malms. 642; R. Glouc. 8841), and Wm. f. Audeline (Gir.
Cam. v. 337; Conq. Ire. 112). Only Athelstan is described
as being thin in person, *corpore deducto* (Wm. Malms. 213).

Leanness of body may be caused by (a) *Sorrow,* cf. Max.
40; (b) *Prison life,* cf. Cur. Mun. 4547; Sed. Sag. 3449, but
after being in prison for a long time, St. Katherine was " swiþe
fat and round," Horst. D. 25. 199; (c) *Penance,* cf. Horst. D.
433; (d) *Unrequited love,* cf. Horst. D. 29. 11; Parton. 6664
(cf. Skeat to Chaucer, Vol. I. p. 548). It may be supposed,
then, that a lean body is not considered beautiful. Indeed of
one fair woman it is stated explicitly that " She was not lene,
but flesly a lyte," Parton. 5161.

§ 18. SHOULDERS.

The shoulders of strong, handsome men must necessarily be
large, thick, and especially broad.[1] Cf. *pectus et humeri dif-
funduntur,* Gir. Cam. VIII. 279; ' þa com þe king of Mede, þe
muchele & þe brade,' La3. 27542; ' brod in þe scholdres,' Havel.
1647; ' schuldres boþe þicke & brade,' Cur. Mun. 7325; Trist.
1556; Ferum. 551, 1072; Iw. & Gaw. 423; Barb. I. 386; Isum.
14; Sc. Leg. 19. 21, 240; Dest. 3966; Lyd. II. 4552; ' byg of
his schuldres,' Dest. Tr. 3760, 3796; ' schuldris ... shapon of
a clene brede,' Dest. Tr. 3823; ' schuldris square & brode,' Lyd.

---

[1] So in the O. Fr. cf. Loubier, *op. cit.* p. 97; Voigt, *op. cit.* p. 60; in the
Germ. cf. Schultz, *op. cit.* I. p. 216. Comp. Chaucer, Rom. Rose. 825; C. T.,
A. 2136; in Philos. p. 85 one of the tokens of a good man is that his
" shuldrys bowe a litel mesurably "; Sec. Sec. pp. 116, 227.

ii. 4575; Horst. C. Misc. 20c. 1448; Troy H. 1084; Grail 13. 649; Guy. B. 4299; 'kurbe schuldris,' Lyd. ii. 4624. The enormous strength of giants is sometimes suggested by the great breadth of the shoulders. Cf. ' four fet in þe face ... & fiften in brede' (Vernagu), Rol. & Vern. 476; ' brade in the scholders,' Mort. Arth. 1094; ' tuo elle in brede, with scholdrys greet,' Oct. S. 926.

The shoulders of women should be ' fair,' well-shaped, white (*shene*), and slightly sloping.[2] Cf. ' Schuft schulders aright,' Alis. A. 186; ' scholdres schaply and schire,' Pist. Sus. 194, 197; ' shuldre ase mon wolde,' Bödd. W. L. x. 28; Erl. Tol. 356; ' Wiþ lowe [3] scholders,' Tars. 15; *Demissi pendent humeri,* Gir. Cam. i. 350. Helen is described,

> With schulders full shaply, shenest of hewe,
> ffull pleasaund & playn, with a plase lawe
> Goyng downe as a goter fro the gorge euyn,   Dest. Tr. 3070.

I have been able to find only one instance of decidedly white shoulders, namely, in the description of Hector. He is struck on the shoulders with a sword and " þeo blod made red þat whyt was are," Troy B. 1413.

Narrow, rough, stooping bent shoulders are ugly. Cf. ' rough y-schuldreod also,' Alis. L. 6813; ' Hir necke is schort, hir schuldres courbe,' Gower, i. 1687. Stooping of the shoulders is also a sign of old age. Cf. Gir. Cam. viii. 279; Horst. D. 47. 238; Horst. A. 3. 224.

§ 19. BREAST: BREASTS.

The breast of an ideal man must be broad, square (quarré, *quadratus*), thick, strong, and hard with brawny muscles. Cf. *pectore quadratus,* Gir. Cam. v. 324 (cf. ' well I-brested,' Conq.

---

[2] So in the Latin, cf. Blümmner, *op. cit.* pp. 22, 34, 40; in the O. Fr. cf. Loubier, *op. cit.* p. 97; Voigt, *op. cit.* p. 60; in the German, cf. Schultz, *op. cit.* i. 216; Weinhold DF. i. 227. Comp. Leahy, " very high, soft and white were her shouldres," i. p. 13.

[3] The word ' lowe' here probably means ' gently sloping.' But in the O. Fr. Loubier records *basses* in the sense of ' broad,' used twice to describe the shoulders of fair women, cf. *op. cit.* p. 97.

The Middle English Ideal of Personal Beauty 113

Ire. 99); Gir. Cam. v. 303 (Conq. Ire. 'brest thyk,' 88) ;
'brustes ful quarreé,' Ferum. 1072; 'brest full square and
mete,' Lyd. II. 4552; Gir. Cam. VIII. 279; 'Brode of his brest,'
Dest. Tr. 3796, 3936, 3775, 3760; Troy H. 1083; Guy. B.
4299; *thoroso pectore,* Wm. Malms. 642 (cf. R. Glouc. ' þikke
of breste,' 8841); Havel. 1648; '*amplo ... pectore,* Trev. VIII.
22; 'large brestid,' Lyd. II. 4611, 4647, 4951; 'A hard brest,'
Dest. Tr. 3967; 'For of bak & of brest al were his bodi sturne,'
Gaw. & Gr. Kn. 143. In descriptions of giants, a broad breast
is a sign of great strength. Cf. 'Hys breste was brode,' Guy.
C. 7761; Guy. B. 7581.

Women. The breast of a beautiful woman should be rather
broad, and as white as snow or as clear as crystal. The breasts
(*mamillae*) must be small, round as a pear or as an apple of
paradise, and as soft as silk to the touch.[1] Cf. *custodia cordis
Quadratur pectus; parva mamilla tumet,* Gir. Cam. I. 350;
'Hir brest . . . Schon schyrer þen snawe þat schedes on hilleȝ;
Gaw. & Gr. Kn. 955. The little hollow in the throat of Helen
just above the breast is perfectly formed,

> The slote of hir slegh brest sleght for to showe,
> As any cristall clere, þat clene was of hewe (Dest. Tr. 3063),

while her whole bosom is as white as foam, and covered with
minute pimples such as are common to healthy skins,

> The brede of hir brest, bright on to loke,
> Was pleasaund & playne pluttide a litull,
> ffresshe and of fyne hew as þe fome clere (Dest. Tr. 3077),

and her pear-like breasts are fair and sweet,

> With two propur pappes as a peire rounde,
> ffetis and faire, of favour full swete (Dest. Tr. 3080).

---

[1] Evidently large breasts are considered ugly. Comp. Chaucer, C. T., A.
3975, 'brestes rounde and hye.' In the German long, hanging breasts are
ugly, cf. Schultz, *op. cit.* I. p. 221. In Old Fr. small breasts, hard as
apples, are beautiful, cf. Gautier, *op. cit.* p. 376. In the English there is
just one description of either hard or soft breasts, namely, in Lydgate's
Reson and Sensuallyte, ed. Sieper, 1643; "Of hir pappis softe as silke."
For the conceit which makes the space between the breasts Cupid's nest, cf.
Ogle, II. 141 f.

8

Cf. further 'with brestis faire & whyte,' Lyd. ii. 4982; 'papes round,' Horst. C. 34. 617; 'hyre tyttes aren an vnder bis As apples two of parays,' Bödd. W. L. v. 58, 74; 'Hire paps were als rounde ywyse, As an appille þate growes in felde,' Horst. B. Misc. 6. 441.[2] Pigeon- or chicken-breasted persons are exceedingly ugly. Cf. *pectore gibboso,* Gir. Cam. iv. 420; 'bouked byfore and byhynde,' Alis. L. 6265; 'Brok-brestede as a brawn with brustils fulle large,' Mort. Arth. 1095.

§ 20. BACK.

The back of a handsome knight should correspond in broadness and strength to the powerful breast. Cf. 'For of bak & of brest were his bodi sturne,' Gaw. & Gr. Kn. 143; 'A hard brest hade þe buerne, & his bak sware,' Dest. Tr. 9342. A fair lady is "Wel shapen both body and bak," Bev. O. 401.

Very ugly is a crooked or a humped back. Cf. 'bouche on bak,' Cur. Mun. 8087; 'bouked byfore and byhynde,' Alis. L. 6265; 'A ful grete bulge opon his bak,' Iw. & Gaw. 307; 'courbe upon his bak,' Gower, v. 956; 'a risyng bak,' Lyd. ii. 4648. A strange people have backs " rughe as a resche " (rush), Alis. L. 4726; and certain giants can find no horses able to carry them, " Ther bakkes and ther belly were so large," Gener. 2155. (Comp. Mabinog. 210).

§ 21. SIDES: WAIST.

The sides of a beautiful woman are tender and soft as silk, white as the fresh morning milk, slender and long,[1] tapering down to a small waist. Cf. 'softe siden,' Marh. fol. 52; 'eyþer

---

[2] The descriptions of women's breasts in the legends are occasioned at the stripping of female saints for torture. A very common form of torture is the tearing away of the breasts with sharp or red-hot instruments, cf. Sc. Leg. 45. 288; 50. 980; Boc. 11. 307; 3. 904 etc.

[1] So in the Latin, cf. Blümmner, *op. cit.* p. 35 in the O. Fr. cf. Voigt,

side softe ase sylk, Whittore þan þe moren mylk,' Bödd. W. L.
LV. 76 (cf. Willms, *op. cit.* p. 27 on *moren*); Horst. C. Misc.
21. 414; Amad. 717; ' Sides seemely sett seemlich long,' Alis.
A. 189; 'Hur sydes long, hur myddyl small,' Erl. Tol. 355.
The sides of men should be as white as the feather of swan,
great, round, and strong,[2] and, as in the case of women, very
long, tapering down to a small waist. Cf. ' Sides þai made blo
& wan, þat er wer white so feþer on swan,' Horn. Ch. 76;
' Rounde sydes,' Dest. Tr. 3822; ' Grete sydes to gripe growen
full sad,' Dest. Tr. 3965; ' Me clupede him uor is stalwardhede
Edmund yrensyde,' R. Glouc. 5939, 6138, 8739; 'Wyþ longe
sydes & middel small,' Ferum. 1073.

As I have already suggested, a long and slender waist is
a criterion of elegance and beauty both in the male and female
form. Cf. ' Wiþ middel smal & wel y-make,' Bödd. W. L. II.
16; Middel ... menskful smal,' Bödd. W. L. x. 31; 'a mete
myddel smal,' Bödd. W. L. v. 73; Ferum. 2199; Launf. M.
944; Launf. R. 439; Erl. Tol. 355; Gower, VI. 786; ' gentil
myddel smal,' Alis. L. 210. If nature denies the desired willowy waist, women, then as now, resort to tight lacing; " kyrlyls
they had of purpyl sendelle, Smalle i-laside syttyig welle,"
Launf. R. 53; Launf. M. 232.[3]

In the description of the Green Knight the breadth of his
back and breast is placed in striking contrast with the smallness
of his waist;

op. cit. p. 60.. Comp. "White as the snow, or as the foam of the wave,
was her side; long was it, slender, and as soft as silk," Leahy, I. p. 13;
"Hir sydes longe, fleshly, smothe, and whyte." Chaucer, Troil. III. 1248.

[2] So in the O. Fr. cf. Loubier, *op. cit.* p. 103. Willms (*op. cit.* p. 21)
quotes from the Pearl, 1137, where the blood drops from the white sides of
the Christ.

[3] Comp. Lanval, 58 f., ' e laciees estreitement en dous bléalz de purpre
bis." For the introduction of corsets or " the whale-bone prison " in the
fourteenth century, cf. Strutt, *op. cit.* II. p. 175. Men also confined their
waists in the time of the Stewarts, cf. Fairholt, *op. cit.* I. p. 286. Cf.
especially the picture of Ann of Denmark, Queen of James the First, Strutt,
Plate CXLII (pp. 145, 175, 266, Vol. II.), and Pl. XCIV.

> For of bak & of brest al were his bodi sturne,
> Bot his wombe & his wast were worthily smale,   Gaw. & Gr. Kn. 143.

Cf. further Ferum. 1072; Lyd. ii. 4624; Conq. Ire. 99; Max 239.

§ 22. ABDOMEN.

The stomachs of women should neither be contracted too much by leanness, nor should they protrude out of measure. Of Eve it is said,

> *Plana superficies ventris succingitur, et nec*
> *Contrahitur macie, nec sine lege tumet,*   Gir. Cam. i. p. 350.

Handsome men, likewise, have small stomachs. Cf. *ventreque substricto.* Gir. Cam. v. 324; 'his wombe ... worthily small,' Gaw. & Gr. Kn. 143.

Exceedingly ugly is a projecting, protuberant stomach.[1] Cf. *ventre praeambulo* (Geof. Archb. of York), Gir. Cam. iv. 420; *carnosa superfluitate ventre turgescens* (Meiler), Gir. Cam. v. 323; 'grete wombe,' (Wm. Rufus), R. Glouc. 8571; Wm. Malms. 607; Trev. vii. 423; 'Ther bakkes and ther belly were soo large, Ther was noo hors of them wold bere the charge' (hideous warriors), Gener. 2155; 'wombes grete' (Magdelene's enemies), Horst. C. 17. 219; 'Of wombe swolle, enbosid with fatnes, þat onneþe he myȝt him silfe sustene' (Polydamas), Lyd. ii. 4664. Henry II. is said to have had an enormous paunch, due rather to nature than to gross feeding (Gir. Cam. v. 303; Conq. Ire. 88), and William the Conqueror also is reported to have been of dignified appearance, tho his protruding belly disfigured an otherwise kingly person (Wm. Malms. 458; R. Glouc. 7731). His last illness was the result of a rupture received while his horse was leaping a ditch (Wm. Malms, 460, 459; R. Glouc. 7788; Trev. vii. 311.

---

[1] Comp. Mabinog. p. 210; Philos. 2661; Sec. Sec. pp. 227, 116. Cf. Voigt, *op. cit.* p. 61.

§ 23. LOINS: HIPS, ETC.

As in the German and Old French, detailed descriptions of the human body below the waist are very rare. This may be due to the fact that those parts are generally covered with rich clothing; but even when the fair one is seen nude, the natural delicacy of the poet prevents him from giving more than information concerning the whiteness of the skin, and the general loveliness of the limbs.

As to the hips of women, they are ' fair,' and not too broad and round. Of Queen Olympias we are told that " Hupes had hue faire & hih was hue þan,' Alis. L. 190. Of a decidedly ugly ·old woman it is said that " Hir body waȝ schort & þik, Hir buttokeȝ bay & brode ' (Gaw. & Gr. Kn. 966), and Chaucer describes the Wife of Bath with "A foot-mantel aboute hir hipes large " (C. T., A. 472).

The ugly Geof. Archb. of York is described with receding loins, *renibus retrogradis* (Gir. Cam. IV. 420), and the terrible giant of Mort. Arth. has loathly, lean flanks with thick haunches like those of a hog (cf. Mort. Arth. 3280, 1100).

Pudenda. The pudenda are mentioned only three times. When the beautiful Floripas is made nude to receive baptism, it is said,

> Was non of hem þat ys flechs ne-raas,
> Noþer kyng, ne baroun, ne non þat was,
> Sche was so fair a þynge   (Ferum. 5888),

which is a less delicate but more realistic way of saying,

> A mains de nos barons est li talens mués,   Fierabras, 6004.

Of Eve we are told,

> *Subsistunt renes, et se moderamine quodam*
> *Amplificant, subeunt ilia pube tenus.*
> *Plena pudore latent Veneris regione pudenda,*
> *Munere naturae digna favore suae,*   Gir. Cam. I. 350.

And finally, of a terrible man-beast monster it is said, " And large was his odd lome þe lenthe of a ȝerde," Alis. C. 4750.

§ 24. LIMBS: BONES.

The limbs of women must be ' lovely,' without fault or blemish, and above all white. Cf. ' lufly of lym,' Horst. C. 13. 111; ' þat rede blod orn a-doun on hire limes so ȝwite,' Horst. B. 29. 124. Hecuba is described, "hor lymes alle dide more decline To schap of man þan to womanhede" (Dest. Tr. 4964), and of an ugly hag it is said, "Hire body gret and nothing smal . . . Sche hath no lith withoute a lak," Gower, I. 1689.

The limbs of men should be ' fair,' well-made, large, strong, long, with enormous muscles, thews and sinews attached to great bones.[1] Cf. ' lymmes bony & sinowy,' Conq. Ire. 188 (cf. Gir. Cam. v. 344) ; ' armes & other lymmes ful bony, more sinowy than fleysly,' Conq. Ire. 100 (cf. Gir. Cam. v. 324; ' In gret bewte of his lymmys ' (Christ), Sc. Leg. III. 665; ' his limes ... faire heo weren and freo ' (Becket), Horst. D. 27. 1181; ' A fairer child neuer i ne siȝ ... Ne non so faire limes hade,' Bev. A. 536; ' It was so feir a creature, as myȝt be on lyve, Of lymys & of fetour,' Beryn. 893; ' Of shap he was semely & feyre, Of lymes large & longe,' Horst. C. Misc. 10. 28; Dest. Tr. 3744; ' lemys full grete,' Dest. Tr. 3805, 3776, 3749; 'limis full brode,' Dest. Tr. 3761; ' his lyndes & his lymes so longe & so grete,' Gaw. & Gr. Kn. 139; 'His lymmes erre lange, his bones gret,' Isum. 247; ' Alle his lymys compact were so clene,' Lyd. III. 1227; ' He is . . . large of lym and lith,' Torr. 2398. Priam is described, "Of hiȝe stature with lymys sklender & longe," Lyd. II. 4781.

Bones. It is not surprising to find that the bones of valiant knights are well-made, large and strong. Cf. *ossa reperta corporis Arthuri . . . grandia fuerunt,* Gir. Cam. VIII. 128; ' wel of bones maked,' Havel. 1646; ' a man of great bones,' Degree P. 444; Guy. C 7911; Bev. A. 4184; Barb. I. 386; ' Of bonys styffe and stronge,' Gregor R. 246; v. 940; A. 666; Rich.

---

[1] Comp. Chaucer, "His limes grete, his braunes harde and stronge," C. T., A. 2135, cf. 1423; "Ful big he was of braun, and eek of bones," C. T., A. 546.

559, 3903; Alis. L. 1740, 2685, 7322; Grail. 13. 652; 'He is so big of bone & blood,' Torr. 1714, 2364; Parton. 7968; 'of bones large and longe,' Parton. 7291; R. Glouc. 8571. Only St. Stephen has small bones, " tobrusede is smale bones," R. Glouc. 6059.

Muscles. Big, strong muscles are also highly appreciated. Cf. ' monnene strengest of maine and of þeauwe,' Laȝ. 6351; 'big senowis,' Dest. Tr. 8794; Lyd. ii. 4943; 'Of brawn & bonys compact be measure,' Lyd. ii, 4815; ' þe mosseles lieȝen wel grete,' Horst. D. 52. 27; ' þe wale thewes þat in þat cors was enclosed,' Alis. C. 2932.

Flesh. However strong and hard the brawn of warriors may be, the flesh of women and children should be tender and as soft as silk. Cf. ' flesh þat tendre was, and swiþe nesh ' (young Havelok), Havel. 2742; ' Softe as selk hee gan hiere fynde,' Parton. 236; Adler. 8; Horst. C. Misc. 21. 416. The flesh of tortured saints is always tender and soft. Cf. ' hyre flesche teyndir & clere,' Sc. Leg. 28. 291; 45. 153; Horst. D. 26. 146; Boc. i. 395; Horst. D. 19. 51; Havel. 216.

In descriptions of powerful warriors, lightness and agility of movement are often mentioned in terms of the highest praise. Cf. 'Gye was bothe stronge and lyght,' Guy. B. 8031; Alis. L. 3891, 4996, 6578; Sow. Bab. 905; Cur. Mun. 6951; Otuel, 829; Lyd. ii. 4855; 'Men that licht and delyuer war,' Barb. x. 61; Lyd. ii. 4638. Various objects of comparison are used to give some idea of this much-praised celerity and quickness of movement.[2] The noble hero is as light as dew, or as a fowl in flight, or, in action of battle, he springs like lightning, or like an arrow from the bow, or like a " sparkle on glede." Cf. ' As liȝt as dew he leyde hem doune,' Launf. M. 607; ' as lyght

---

[2] For many other citations cf. Regel, Spruch und Bild im Laȝamon, *Anglia*, i. p. 232 ff.; Wülfing, Das Bild und die Bildiche Verneinung im Laud Troy Book, *Anglia*, xxviii, p. 33; Klaeber, Das Bild bei Chaucer (1893); Heise, *op. cit.* p. 69. The comparison 'like a sparkle on glede,' seems to be particularly English. Cf. Regel's comparative citations from O. Fr. *Angl.* i. p. 232.

Als a fowl es to the flyght,' Iw. & Gaw. 1302, 629; 'He loked as layt so ly3t,' Gaw. & Gr. Kn. 199; 'He was lyght als lefe one tree,' Rol. & Ot. 996; 'Owt he sprang As fyr Offe brond,' Grail. 13. 543; 'Als arewe of bowe forth he sprang,' Alis. L. 5538; 'He sprang owt as sperkulle on glede,' Oct. N. 1465, 961, 1034; Tars. 194; Isum. C. 458; Pier. Lang. 7122; La3. 21481, 23507; Havel. 90; Gol. & Gaw. 978; Sow. Bab. 205; and when Alexander has a new horse brought to him in battle, he "leop on his rugge, So a goldfynch doth on the hegge," Alis. L. 782.

Here may be mentioned those circumlocutions or paraphrases which may mean merely 'entirely,' or may refer sometimes to the personal appearance in general. Cf. 'He is as big of *bone & blood,*' Torr. 577; 'þe Normandes gude of blode & bone,' Rol. & Ot. 706, 891, 984, 1295, 1409, 1563, 1534; 'a stronge man of blode and bone,' Bon. Flor. 14; Eger. & Gr. 499; Cur. Mun. 27615; Am. & Am. 142; Torr. 2555; Tars. 577; Pier Lang. 985; Am. & Am. 344; Gowth. A. 550, 6328; Torr. 1714, 2364, 112; '*breyn & blod,*' Bon. Flor. 1942. (b), *Flesh and fell.* Cf. 'She was fayre of flessh and felle,' Gowth. 33; Emar. 306; 'full fayre of flesche & fell' (knights), Rol. & Ot. 881; Emar. 735; Horst. D. 17. 14; 39, 157; R. Glouc. 5815; Thos. Ercel. C. 507; Bev. A. 311, 3344; Grail. 21. 314; 'Neuer man of flesche ne felle nas so strong,' Bev. A. 14; Cur. Mun. 584, 15643; Rol. & Ot. 96; Tars. 770; Cur. Mun. p. 987. 156, 19961, 23603: 'Nas neuer 3ut so lodly man ymad of flehs & felle' (Alagolafre), Ferum. 4439. (c), *Flesh and bone.* Cf. 'The feyrest woman... That myghth be made of flessche and bonys,' Orph. 51; Ferum. 5885; 'so semely of fleshe and bone,' Squyr. 709, 1085; 'Nis þer non so bald, Ymade of flesche no ban' (warrior), Trist. 997; 'Thou art strong in flesch and bones,' Rich. 5445; 'A lodluker damme þan sche was on... of fleche & bon, Neuere no man ne y-say' (giantess), Ferum. 4665. (d), *Flesh and blood.* Cf. 'Hardy is his flesch and blod,' Alis. L. 3009. (e), *Fell and bone.* Cf. 'so fair creature nas non Ase was þis maide forthward of felle noþer of bon,' Horst.

D. 29. 5. (f), *Body and bones.* Cf. ' þat doȝthy of body and bon,' Gowth. A. 450.[3]

§ 25. ARMS.

The arms of a noble knight must be long, great, round, and especially strong and sinewy.[1] The arms of Wm. the Conqueror are so strong that he can easily shoot a bow which no one else can bend; *fuit . . . roboris ingentis in lacertis, ut magno saepe spectaculo fuerit quod nemo ejus arcum tenderet, quem ipse admisso equo pedibus nervo extento sinuaret,* Wm. Malms. 458; Trev. VII. 314; R. Glouc. 7733. Duke Meiler has arms bony and more sinewy than fleshy; *brachiis . . . ossosis, plus nervositatis habentibus quam carnositatis,* Gir. Cam. v. 327 (Conq. Ire. 100). Cf. further, ' armes stronge,' Laȝ. 30095; Isum. 14; ' stithe in his armys,' Dest. Tr. 3795; Gir. Cam. v. 303 (Conq. Ire. 88); ' armys gret,' Lyd. II. 4574, 6311; ' armys large and rounde,' Lyd. II. 4625; ' big of his armys,' Dest. Tr. 3966, 3775, 9475; ' armes long,' Trist. 1556 (comp. Chaucer, ' armes rounde and longe,' C. T., A. 2136); ' Grete armys in the gripe growen full rounde,' Dest. Tr. 3761.

The arms of lovely women should be small but plump, and long.[2] Cf. *Parturiunt humeri procerae brachia formae,* Gir. Cam. I. 350; ' White hond & long arm,' Arth. & Merl. 745 (and note); ' eyþer arm an elne long,' Bödd. W. L. v. 52;

---

[3] Here may be mentioned such expressions as "hardy blood," Alis. L. 5521; "a-wondrith al my blod," Alis. L. 1407; for sorrow "Al chaunged was hire blod," Sev. Sag. 466. I have found no descriptions of veins, but Strutt mentions the custom of painting them blue, cf. *op. cit.* II. 235. Cf. also Sec. Sec. p. 229.

[1] So in the O. Fr. cf. Loubier, *op. cit.* p. 98; Gautier, *op. cit.* p. 206. Comp. Sec. Sec. "Whenne þe armes rechyn so farre, þat þe hondes ateigne to þe knees, bytokyns hardynesse, and prowesse, with largesse," p. 117. Cf. further *ibid.* p. 235; Philos. p. 84.

[2] So in the Germ. cf. Weinhold, *op. cit.* DF. I. 227; Schultz, *op. cit.* I. 217; in the O. Fr. cf. Gautier, *op. cit.* p. 376. In the Latin and German the arms of women should be as white as snow or as ivory, cf. Blümmner, *op. cit.* pp. 32, 34, 40; Ogle III. 468. Comp. Leahy, VI. p. 13, "Each of her two arms was as white as the snow of a single night."

'Hir armys were auenaund & abill of shap, Large of a lenght, louely to shewe,' Dest. Tr. 3073 (comp. Chaucer, ' armes, every lith Fattish, flesshy, not greet therwith,' Duchess, 953) ; ' Armes smalle,' Parton. 5162, 6180 (comp. Chaucer, Troil. III. 1247, and cf. Ogle III. 463) ; 'well ischaped armes,' Alis. L. 186; ' Wiþ armes . . . ase mon wolde,' Bödd. W. L. x. 28 ; ' armes . . . Fayrer myght none bee,' Erl. Tol. 356.

Ugly arms are rarely mentioned. Deformed men are described with " her armes hery wiþ blak hide " Cur. Mun. 8085 (comp. MS. Göt. ' harplid hide ' ; MS. Fair. ' rungilt hide '), a loathly giant has " Ruyd armes as an ake," Mort. Arth. 1096, and St. Martin after much fasting has " Armes smale and lene," Horst. D. 64. 218.

§ 26.   HAND: FINGERS: FIST

The hands of charming women are ' fair,' beautifully formed, sweet as violet, and deft. Cf. ' fair fot and hond' Arth. & Merl. 743 'Hondes hendely wrought helplich swete,' Alis. A. 187; Parton. 5162 ; ' Hyr handes were swete as vyolet,' Bev. O. 401; ' hondes slye,' Horn. Ch. 435 ; ' rekene ase regnas,' Bödd. W. L. I. 42 (" schnell bei der hand," Bödd.).

An especial mark of beauty is the whiteness of the hands,[1]

---

[1] So in the Latin, cf. Blümmner, *op. cit.* pp. 22, 35, 40; in the O. Fr. cf. Loubier, *op. cit.* p. 99; Gautier, *op. cit.* p. 376; Ott, *op. cit.* p. 7; and in the German, cf. Schultz, *op. cit.* I. p. 217; Weinhold DF. I. p. 227: and in the Old Norse, cf. Weinhold AL. p. 32. For The 'White Hand' of Shakespeare's Heroines, cf. M. P. Tilly, *Sewanee Review,* Vol. XIX. p. 207. Ogle III (*Sewan. Rev.* XX. p. 459) presents many other citations from 16th century English literature, and by comparative quotations shows that the ' white hand ' is a literary conceit which may be traced back thru Old French and Italian to Classical times. Such conceits probably originated in the Alexandrian schools of rhetoric (p. 468). Cf. Buckhardt, *op. cit.* p. 66, Vol. I. for the Italian. Comp. " her fingers long and of great whiteness," Leahy I. p. 13. In the English and Scottish Ballads " A milk-white hand is mentioned wherever possible " . . . even men have the conventional ' lily hands,' Mead B. p. 326. For other citations from Mid. Eng. cf. Willms, *op. cit.* p. 21.

together with long, slender fingers.[2] Hands and fingers are sometimes white as snow, white as whale's bone (ivory), milk-white or lily-white. Cf. *Producunt niveas brachia longa manus,* Gir. Cam. I. 350; 'White hond,' Arth. & Merl. 745; 'Ysonde . . . Wiþ þe white hand,' Trist. 2650, 2677, 3046; 'Ysonde wiþ hand schene,' Trist. 2660; 'whitte hondeȝ,' Mort. Arth. 3262; Gower, VI. 779; Grail. 24. 36; 'lik As Snow they weren so whit,' Grail. 25. 336; 'When y byholde vpon hire hond, þe lylie white lef in lond best heo mihte beo,' Bödd. W. L. v. 49 ; ' Hur hondys whyte as wallys bone, Wyth longe fyngurs, that fayre schone, Hur nayles bryght of blee,' Erl. Tol. 358; 'with her milke white honde,' Eger. & Gr. 301, 252. Twice we find men presented with white hands (cf. Horst. C. p. 501. 1. 129; Arth. & Merl. 8266). Other beautiful women have "fyngeris smale," Lyd. IV. 594; Orf. 101; 'small hondus, and fyngurs longe,' Bev. M. 401; and Helen has also fingernails as white as a turnip;

> Hir hondus fetis & faire, with fingurs full small,
> With nailes at the neþer endes as a nepe white, (Dest. Tr. 3075),

with which may be compared Chaucer's Duchesse (954),

> Right whyte handes, and nayles rede.[3]

As for men, their hands should be large—with long fingers and sharp fingernails—strong and powerful in battle. Cf. 'longe honden,' Alis. L. 2001; ' þe hondene fair and longe fingres, fairore ne miȝten none beo,' Horst. D. 27. 1180; 'it was red rowed to see, with fingars more than other three,' Eger. & Gr. 1181, 1217; 'his nayles scharpe,' Horn. 247; 'Aelc finger an his hond, scharp stelene brond,' Laȝ. 18864; 'With smale handes And fyngres longe, And therto gret strengthe Amonge,' Grail. 13. 653; 'hondis strong,' Lyd. II. 4625; 'He wolde esi-

---

[2] Comp. Leahy, I. p. 13; Sec. Sec. pp. 117, 235; Philos. p. 85. In the Latin and Old Fr. beautiful fingers are rosy cf. Blümmner, *op. cit.* pp. 202, and Loubier, *op. cit.* p. 100, but I have not found it so in the Mid. Eng.

[3] Comp. "her nails were beautiful and pink " (Leahy, I. p. 13), and the custom of staining the nails pink among the Irish, "No more my nails with pink I stain," Leahy, I. p. 100.

liche wiþ his hondes folde and bende foure hors schoon at ones'
(Charles the Great), Trev. vi. 255.

Probably entirely metaphorical are the expressions; 'þe
harde hond,' Ferum. 455, 3186; 'mon of myghty hond,' Alis.
L. 97, 631, 3867; 'felle honde,' Alis. L. 2078; 'ful manly of
his hande,' Gener. 1930; 'knyghtes douhty of handes,' Pier
Lang. 353; 'stark hande,' Sc. Leg. 33. 947; 'wyght of hys
honde,' Guy. B. 8879; 'stalward man he was of hand,' Cur.
Mun. 24767; 'Hardi of honde,' Avow. Arth. i. 11; 'heuy
hond,' Ferum. 5555.

Fist. Highly appreciated is the fist that is large, strong and
square (Barb. iii. 581), and admirable is the blow from it which
breaks the neck of the enemy so that he rises no more (Guy. B.
5476; Gol. & Gaw. 106; Guy. B. 5083; 8868; Troy H. 1636;
Troy B. 1948; Ferum. 2248), or causes the eyes to fly from
their sockets (Ferum. 2248; Gener. 1482), or the teeth from
the bone (Ferum. 5649, 5795). To have the brains of the
enemy cleave about the fist of the hero after a mighty stroke
is especially admirable (cf. Ferum. 1900).

Deformed, crooked hands are ugly.[4] Cf. 'Also stif ase ani
hard bord hire hond bi-cam . . . And þe hond was . . . fur-
crokeed,' Horst. D. 63. 343, 351; 'hondis al for-skramyd,'
Beryn. 2381, 2514. Nails allowed to grow long so as to resemble claws are decidedly ugly.[5] Cf. 'nayles growen and all
for-fare,' Parton. 6655; 'Scharpe clawyde & longe nayled'
(Devil), Horst. C. Misc. 12. 295.

§ 27.   LEGS.

The legs of a good knight are long, straight, strong and firm
in battle, with thighs brawny and thick. Cf. 'Sturne stif on

---

[4] So are black hands, cf. " Blacker were her two hands than the blackest
iron covered with pitch," Mabinog. p. 209. In the Old Norse calloused
hands with stiff, short fingers are ugly, cf. Weinhold, AL. p. 33.

[5] Comp. Chaucer, " His nayles lik a briddes clawes were," C. T., B. 3366.
For manner of cutting the nails in Italian, cf. Buckhardt, *op. cit.* 67.

þe stryþþe on stalworþ schonkeȝ,' Gaw. & Gr. Kn. 846; 'stal-
worth shankes,' Chev. Ass. 326; 'his shankes full seemlye
shone,' Eger. & Gr. 957; 'His thik þrawen þyȝeȝ,' Gaw. & Gr.
Kn. 578; 'leel theghes,' Dest. Tr. 8800; 'With grete thyes,'
Grail. 13. 648; Gir. Cam. VIII. 129. Giraldus Cambrensis
also mentions the English custom, not known among the Irish,
of artificially stretching the thighs of young children; *Non
enim obstetrices aquae calentis beneficio . . . tibias extendunt,*
Gir. Cam. v. 150.

Knights are also long-coupled, i. e. the fork where the thighs
come together is wide and 'long,' so as to permit a firm seat in
the saddle. This forkedness is expressed by the borrowed Old
French word *forcheure*.[1] Cf. 'a man of gret stature, & ful
brod in þe scholdres, was a long man in forchure,' Ferum. 550;
'XII fote long, Wyde and long in heore forchur,' Alis. L. 6315;
'forchures swithe wide,' Alis. L. 4995.

The nether limbs of women should be well-formed, with
thighs smooth, soft and inviting to the touch, and as white as
milk.[2] Cf. 'þeȝes, legges, fet ant al ywroht wes of þe beste,'
Bödd. W. L. x. 33; 'Hur þies all þorou-oute þristliche ischape,
With likand legges louely too sene,' Alis. A. 192; 'This white
leggys,' Gener. 4402, 4408. Of Eve we are told,

> *Invitat femorum caro lactea, lubrica, mollis,*
> *Lumina, lac, glacies, mollitiesque manus;*
> *Corporis egregii gemmae stant crura columnae,* Gir. Cam. I. 350.

On the other hand, when the Fairy Queen is transformed, she
is hideous with "Hir a schanke blake"[3] (Thos. Ercel. 135),
Goliath has "leggis longe" (Cur. Mun. 7447), and a terrible
beast-man-giant, "laith leggis & longe," Alis. C. 4748.

---

[1] For full discussion of the word cf. Loubier, *op. cit.* p. 105; Voigt, *op. cit.*
pp. 61, 49. In O. Fr. women with great forcheures are ugly.

[2] Comp. "Smooth and white were her thighs; her knees were round and
firm and white; her ankles were as straight as the rule of a carpenter,"
Leahy, I. p. 13.

[3] Comp. "her legs were large and bony. And her figure was very thin
and spare, except for her feet and her legs which were of huge size,"
Mabinog. 210.

Unshapely, crooked, and distorted legs or thighs are ugly. Cf. *tibiis tortis,* Gir. Cam. IV. 420; ' Crompled knees,' Cur. Mun. 8087; ' With schankeʒ unschaply, schowande to-gedyrs,' Mort. Arth. 1099; ' he was hepehalt,' Gower, v. 957; Sc. Leg. 7. 124. From Chaucer's description of the. Reve we may conclude that small, lean, pipe-stem legs are objects of derision;

> Ful long were his legges, and full lene,
> Y-lyk a staf, ther was no calf y-sene,   C. T., A. 591.

§ 28.   FEET.

Definite and detailed descriptions of beautiful feet are rare. The poet generally contents himself with saying that they are ' fair,' well-shaped, or wrought in the best manner possible; but that small feet are especially characteristic of beautiful women can scarcely be doubted.[1]   After the body of Eve has been described in detail, it is said,

> *Corporis egregii gemmae stant crura columnae,*
> *Mobile fundamen pes brevis ima tenet,*   Gir. Cam. I. 350.

Cf. further, ' fair fot & hand,' Arth. & Merl. 743; *ibid.* p. 678; ' a louely mouth and fayre fete,' Bev. O. 402; ' þe fairest feete þat euer freke kende,' Alis. A. 193; ' þeʒes, legges, fet ant al ywroht wes of þe beste,' Bödd. W. L. x. 33; ' Shee was well shapen of foote & hand,' Triam. P. 652; Parton. Frag. 49. Queen Olympias has " ton tidily wrought " (Alis. A. 194), and one of the characteristics of an ideal woman is " that sche hath a litel heile " (Gower v. 2484).

As to men, one fair knight is described as being " well-fauored of ffoote & hand " (Degree p. 77), and Salomé has " Plate feet and longe honden," Alis. 2001.   (I cannot imagine

---

[1] In the O. Fr. and Germ. delicately arched feet are highly prized, cf. Voigt, *op. cit.* p. 61; Schultz, *op. cit.* p. 219. Comp. Weinhold DF. I. p. 228; Weinhold AL. p. 31. In the Latin beautiful feet are described as being snow-white, cf. Blümmner, *op. cit.* pp. 35, 40. Comp. " Her feet were slim and as white as the ocean's foam," Leahy I. p. 13.

why the handsome knight, Salomé, should be given flat feet. Cf. Halliwell, *Plat-footed,* splay-footed.).

Immensely large feet are, of course, ugly. Cf. *in modico corpore pes immensus,* Gir. Cam. IV. 420; ' His an fot was more than othir two,' Alis. L. 6815; ' hee was large of ffoote & hand, As any man within the Land ' (dwarf), Degree P. 654. The cannibal monster of Mort. Arth. (1098) is shovel-footed, and scaly; " Schovelle fotede was þat schalke, and schaylande hyme semyde "; and a strange people have one foot so large that they protect themselves from the sun and rain with it (Alis. L. 4975; comp. Mabinog. 210).